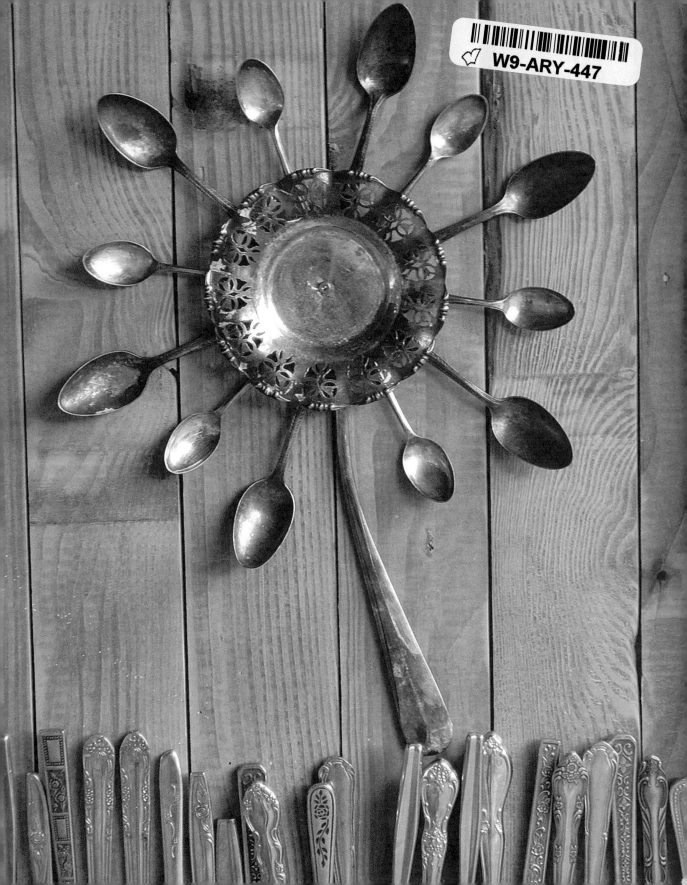

"*Bountiful Baby Purées* is filled with amazing gems for families—including recipes, tips on eating locally and organically, and suggestions on how to live simply and sustainably. This is a wonderful book!"

—RACHEL LINCOLN SARNOFF, C.E.O. and Executive Director, Healthy Child Healthy World

"*Bountiful Baby Purées* provides delicious, baby-approved recipes alongside enough mouthwatering pictures that your whole family will be begging you to make more! Anni Daulter takes us on a baby-inspired culinary journey using only the freshest and purest ingredients around. The recipes range from the simplest of purées for beginner eaters to downright mouthwatering finger foods your entire family will enjoy. It's great to finally find a baby food book that covers it all: fast, affordable, fresh recipes that are yummy enough for children of all ages!"

—MARTHA LEE, mom-blogger for PaulaDeen.com

"Whether you have a baby or want to be 'babied,' this cookbook is filled with real, fresh ingredients blended into the most amazing recipes by hip author-mom Anni Daulter."

—KATHY KAEHLER, celebrity trainer, spokesperson, and author of *Mom Energy*

Bountiful Baby Purées

Create Nutritious Meals for Your Baby with Wholesome Purées Your Little One Will Adore

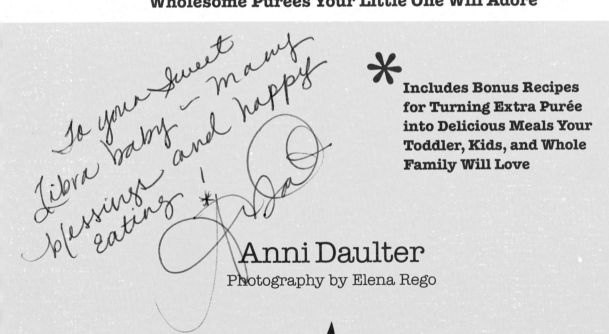

To your sweet Libra baby — many blessings and happy eating!

* **Includes Bonus Recipes for Turning Extra Purée into Delicious Meals Your Toddler, Kids, and Whole Family Will Love**

Anni Daulter

Photography by Elena Rego

FAIR WINDS
PRESS
BEVERLY, MASSACHUSETTS

First published in the USA in 2012 by
Fair Winds Press, a member of
Quayside Publishing Group
100 Cummings Center
Suite 406-L
Beverly, MA 01915-6101
www.fairwindspress.com

16 15 14 13 12   1 2 3 4 5

ISBN: 978-1-59233-516-9

Digital edition published in 2012
eISBN: 978-1-61058-408-1

Library of Congress Cataloging-in-Publication Data available

Cover design by Rita Sowins/Sowins Design
Book design by Rita Sowins/Sowins Design
All photography by Elena Rego with the exception of the following:
Denne Boring/www.etsy.com/shop/DenneAlise, 20 (bottom, left)
Cari Ellen Hermann/www.cariellen.com, 87
Alexandra DeFurio/www.defuriophotography.com, 11; 183
Tnah Louise/www.bellafacciafoto.com, 60; 64 (top, left); 102 (bottom, left)
Gina Sabatella/www.sabatellafoto.com, 6 (top, left); 15; 18 (top); 45; 62 (bottom, right);
   68; 89; 105 (right)
Adam Ziglar/www.ziglarphoto.com, 1
Food styling by Anni Daulter, www.deliciousgratitude.com

Printed and bound in China

✳ Dedication ✳

To my whole family for all of their constant love and support.
To my husband Tim, I love you and appreciate your support more
than you will ever know. To Zoe for teaching me patience
and creativity, to Lotus for teaching me about pure sweet beauty,
to Bodhi for teaching me about fun and laughter, and to River for
teaching me about trust and giving.

To all the babies and families who will be fed from the love of their
parents the recipes in these pages. May your culinary journeys
be filled with flavor, adventure, and love. ~Anni

To my Jon Brown, your consistent, steady presence and support
throughout this little whirlwind project was the anchor that kept me
on track. I love you big. ~Elena

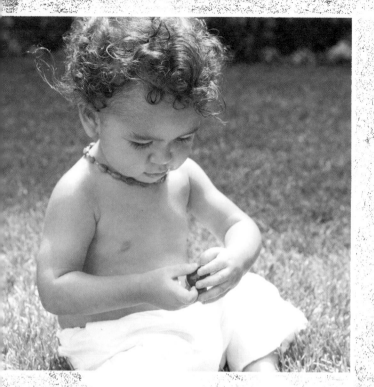
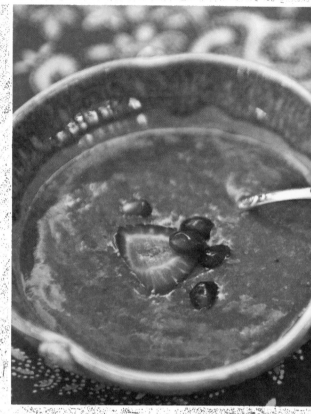
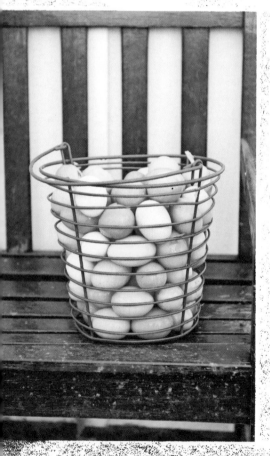
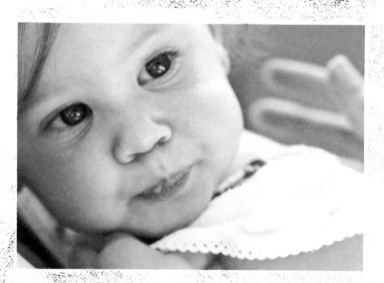
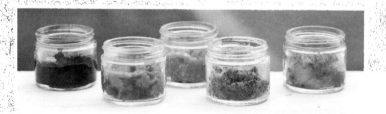

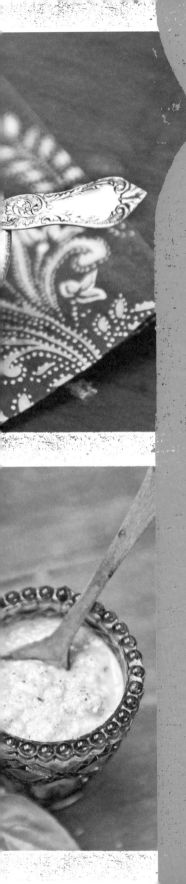

contents

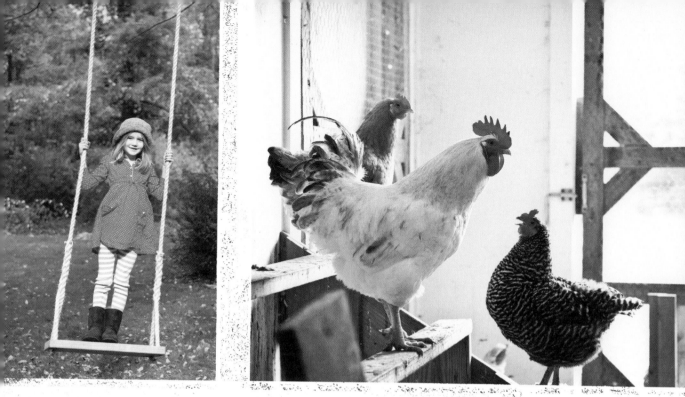

foreword

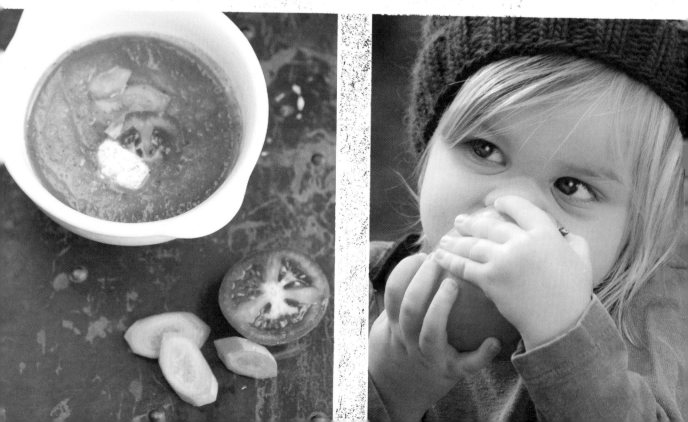

Nourishment. Food. Love. When it comes to nourishing our children, giving love through quality, delicious food is *the* goal, and there is evidence to support this theory. One could offer statistics, for instance, about how organic whole foods contain more nutrients and fewer toxins than conventional foods, thus helping a child's body grow more efficiently and powerfully. Or one could point to how variety in tastes, smells, textures, and colors help children develop more robust senses. Additionally, one could highlight the importance of family interaction around food and the dining experience from baby's earliest days.

There isn't a mom out there who doesn't want to do these things for her child—and herself. Yet there are the issues—the implementation challenges—that so often make what one knows and wants seem more difficult. Families feel stuck and challenged and end up using shortcuts that they might not truly want to.

In walks Anni Daulter, with love, compassion, and years of knowledge and practical solutions. In this book, Anni shows moms how to stay the desired course—to feed baby and family foods that nourish fully. With helpful suggestions and clearly stated reasons why quality food matters, Anni brings you back to the goal, showing that issues can be addressed, one meal at a time.

As a dietitian working with moms everywhere, I am thrilled to introduce you all to *Bountiful Baby Purées*. Use it as a tool, along with Anni's other books, to help fill your mom arsenal and to help nourish your children, your family, and yourself each and every day.

Ashley Koff, R.D.
Author of *Mom Energy: A Simple Plan to Live Fully Charged*
www.AshleyKoffRD.com

introduction

As a mom, I know how important it is to make sure your kids are getting the best nutrition possible, and starting off right just makes things go a lot smoother. Everyone wants to eat fresh delicious foods, even your baby, which is why putting in the time to prepare homemade baby food is a gift you give your child that will last a lifetime. Passing along family cooking, eating, and eco-friendly traditions are priceless and go a long way in supporting a healthy lifestyle. I want this book to be a trusted resource for you to turn to when feeding your whole family foods that you feel good about. I know how personal feeding your baby is to you and how worried parents get when their baby doesn't eat something they should or does eat something they shouldn't. I want to try to help ease some of your concern with tips and ideas and simple recipes to help you give your baby a fresh, healthy start.

I believe food traditions come from an understanding and appreciation of where our food comes from and how it's grown and processed. When parents possess this basic knowledge, they can find ways to pass along important information to their children as they start solid foods and continue down the path of choosing foods for themselves one day. After all, we parents do all of this work so our babies and children will grow into healthy beings that hopefully make sound nutritional choices for themselves, and to do that, they need the tools. Babies eat what we give them, kids eat what they are used to, and adults eat what they like. As parents, we can help shape this trajectory in ways that support healthy bodies and a healthy environment.

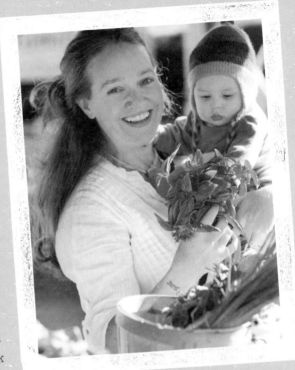

Bountiful Baby Purées is a book that invites you to cook seasonally for your baby by using local, fresh, and organic ingredients. But in the spirit of bounty, I wanted to give you even more. As a conscious-minded mama, I wanted to write a cookbook that would give you those fresh ideas for cooking for your baby but also offer you tips on how to incorporate those wonderful purées and baby foods into your family meals. For those of you with multiple children, like me, this book is a goldmine full of goodies. What I have found is that when you make a bunch of food for your baby, so much of it can go to waste because she often cannot (or doesn't care to) eat it all. Being able to utilize your purées in your family meals will save you time, effort, and money, and it is a great way to incorporate healthy additions to your meals, saving those precious leftover baby purées! I like my cookbooks to somehow cross the age barriers and be suitable for all family members, as I truly believe that everyone, including babies, should be able to take part in the family food table. So explore, exchange, and share these 2-in-one recipes, while supporting your new baby and growing family throughout all the seasons of your life.

With gratitude,

Anni

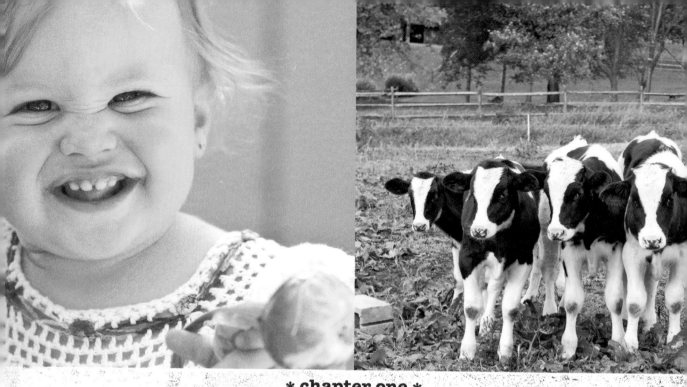

the basics

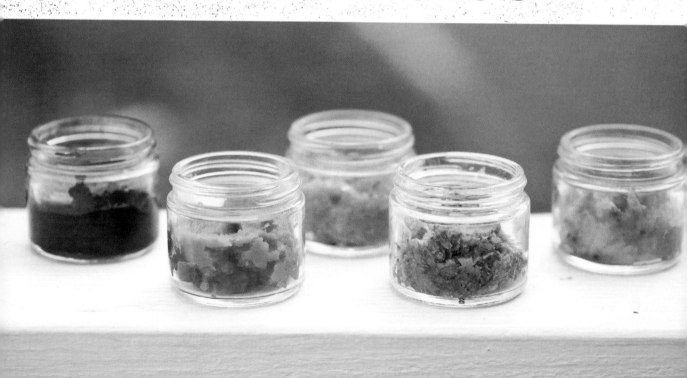

Feeding a brand new baby can seem intimidating, but remember that babies are just little people, and these first bites are just that—little bites. It is important to keep this in mind because all babies are different, and some start earlier than others when it comes to eating solid foods. Boys tend to start eating solid foods earlier and want more than girls, but this is not always the case, of course. Because babies are human beings, there are no set rules we can adhere to for every child. We must listen to them, follow their cues, and trust the process. If you are feeling anxious about food, so will your baby. Likewise, if you are relaxed and excited about food, your child is likely to follow your cues.

Babies tend to be ready for these first tastes of food around six months old, when they are sitting up on their own, and showing interest. Please do not start your baby eating solids before six months old. They do not need it, and their digestive tracts are not formed well enough to process it.

When the magical day finally comes, offer your baby solid food taste tests, offer small bites at a time, and never force your baby to eat. Babies have a natural gag reflex, and when they are starting to try foods, they may use that from time to time. This does not usually mean they are choking, so try not to panic. Simply go to Baby and check for any larger pieces of food that may have slipped through your purée process.

Whether your baby is sitting on your lap or in a high chair when she is trying foods, make sure she is a part of the family table. Including your baby is critical to forming healthy food traditions around the table.

Milk: Where It's At!

The first year of a baby's life should be all about the breast milk. Breast milk is the very best choice for your baby and is what I call the most natural super-food she will ever have. It's chock-full of necessary antibodies that build up your baby's immune system and support her growing body (keeping this in mind should help you sleep at night, especially if you have a baby that does not take to solid foods right away).

Solids are a supplement to the breast milk during that first year of life and should not replace it. Some babies do not start eating solids until around ten or eleven months, and as long as they are getting the milk they need, they are fine. Breastfeed your baby as long as you like—the World Health Organization (WHO) advises breastfeeding to "two years of age or beyond." There is no perfect solid food anywhere that will give your baby all the nutrition that your breast milk does, so give your baby all they want. If your baby is bottle-fed, make sure to choose an organic variety that is full of the most natural ingredients possible.

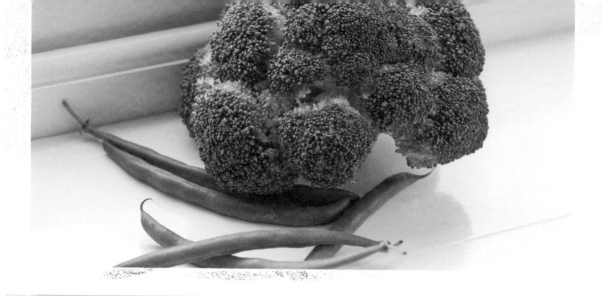

Best First Foods

Do not start your baby on rice cereal. In the past, the majority of pediatricians recommended rice cereal mixed with breast milk or formula as a first food. Today, many pediatricians advise parents to start with fresh, puréed, single-ingredient fruits and veggies. Babies do not need iron fortified processed cereals as long as they are breastfeeding. Your mama's milk provides them with enough nutrients to help them grow, gain weight and build strong immune systems.

When you do start introducing grains, use whole grains, such as millet, whole grain oats, quinoa, and amaranth. Cook and mix these whole grains with your breast milk or one of your purées when you begin this introduction (usually between seven and eight months). Unless you have a history of allergies in your family, you also do not need to try one food at a time and wait in between feedings. These first fruits and vegetables (see box at right) are very low allergens and almost no one is allergic to them, but if your baby is allergic, you will know it by the red rash that forms around his mouth. What this means is that you can mix and match foods right out of the gate.

Keeping your foods fresh and organic is important because these first bites are going directly into your baby's pure system. We want to support a healthy start, and produce that has not been sprayed with dangerous chemicals is the way to go with a baby's sensitive tummy.

Essential Cooking Equipment for Purées and Family Meals

To make baby food, it's helpful to own a steamer, a blender or food processor, and baking sheets. You will also need airtight glass jars. Small mason jars work well. There are fancy baby-food makers out there, but these few basics are all you really need to steam and purée food.

Some of my favorite cooking must-haves to make the family meals include the following:

> Cast iron skillets and pots
> Tabletop mixer
> Tabletop grill

> Slow cooker
> Panini press
> Waffle maker

Don't Hide the Goods!

Hiding vegetable purées in child-friendly food so that they are more palatable to kids is all the rage, but that is not what this book is about. In fact, I encourage you to be open about adding vegetables to your purées, and to your family's meals as well. Involve your kids as helpers in the kitchen so they see exactly what is being put into the food they are eating.

I do not subscribe to hiding food in food; rather, I believe in teaching children about eating healthfully, growing foods, and living simply and sustainably so we all have an earth to enjoy. With this knowledge, children have a healthy awareness of what they put into their bodies and why. Hiding vegetables in other foods makes them mysterious and something taboo. In my house, vegetables are revered—almost honored—because of their deliciousness, price, and how easy they are to grow ourselves. Trust me when I say that children appreciate your honesty, and tricking them into eating healthy food does not establish good eating habits for the future. This is a quick fix to a growing problem in the United States: our children do not eat well, and it is because of convenient fast food and busy lives.

If you want to establish healthy eating for your kids from the start, don't hide the goods!

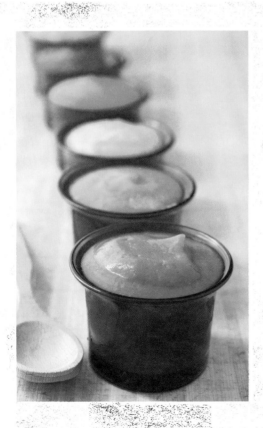

∗ BEST FIRST FRUITS ∗

These first three fruits are great when you are on the go. Just bring them raw and grab a fork and a little wooden bowl to mash.

> Bananas
> Avocados
> Papayas
> Apples
> Pears
> Plums

∗ BEST FIRST VEGGIES ∗

> Peas
> Butternut squash
> Sweet potatoes
> Green beans
> Yellow potatoes
> Carrots
> Broccoli

Double-Duty Recipes to Save You Time

This book has plenty of great ideas for purées and equally exciting family recipes to choose from. In my effort to help parents in the kitchen, every baby purée in this book has a corresponding family-friendly recipe that uses that purée—look for these at the end of each chapter. A small baby can only eat so much, and there is likely to be a surplus of any purées you make, so being able to use the leftovers in creative ways is not only fun, but healthy for your whole family.

Making Mealtime Special

If you value family mealtimes (and I'm sure you do), then so will your children, and including your baby in this process will help her become a part of the family rhythm early on. Setting up a daily rhythm is important so that children and babies know what to expect. This gives them comfort and brings the family together while creating food traditions for them to carry throughout their lives.

Tips for Mealtime Success

In our fast paced lives, we have somehow lost the concept that food is not just about the actual food. It's about the connection, the time spent enjoying every bite, laughing, talking, and sharing. Our families need this time together.

Following are some tips for ensuring mealtime is both fun and restorative for all members of your family.

* CREATE A RHYTHM *

Why is this important? Because offering little ones rhythm brings them a warm sense of understanding of what is happening in their lives, and they thrive off of predictability. This might sound boring to an adult, but children need to know how their days will flow. It offers them a sense of internal peace. This is true for babies and children. If you have multiple children, you can assign them little jobs here and there so that they know what they are responsible for to make the family meals happen. These are simple tasks like carrying the cups to set the table or laying out the napkins and forks and bringing their dishes to the sink after dinner. You might even consider a meal routine, which could ease your creative burdensome.

For example, you could choose purées and meals from this book that support the family cooking rhythms that follow.

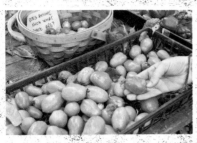

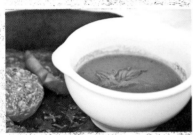

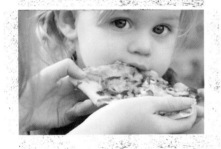

MONDAY: VEGETABLE DISH DAY

Every Monday night, get creative with your veggies. Make meals inspired by your local seasonal fare or your weekly community-supported agriculture (CSA) pick-up.

TUESDAY: PASTA AND PROTEIN

Every Tuesday, create a dish that includes some sort of pasta and meat or other form of protein if you are vegetarian.

WEDNESDAY: SOUP DAY

Every Wednesday, prepare a different soup and serve with fresh grain bread and greens.

THURSDAY: BEANS

Every Thursday night, introduce a different dish made with a variety of beans.

FRIDAY: HOMEMADE PIZZA NIGHT!

Keep Fridays fun with pizza. This is a fun way to be creative and include the kids in the preparation, because everyone can, make her own pizzas with toppings based on her likes.

SATURDAY AND SUNDAY: OPEN

Keep Saturday and Sunday open for your own creations.

✳ KEEP IT CLEAN ✳

Keeping your kitchen clean and organized can help your children learn the value of food care. We want to respect the food environment with which we feed our bodies, and keeping it clean reminds us to be reverent and appreciative of what we have. It's is also a lot more fun to cook in a clean kitchen than a dirty one!

✳ SAY NO TO FIGHTING IN THE KITCHEN ✳

This has been a long-standing rule in my house, and I hope that you adopt it as well. I believe that our food holds not only the nutritional value to feed us, but a spiritual value that nourishes our souls. Everyone has a favorite dish their mom or dad made for them when they were kids, and even if you have had better lasagna at a fancy Italian restaurant, it's not your mama's! This is because although the fancy chef appreciates your business, he does not love you the way your mama does. When you cook for your family, you put your heart in it, and you can taste love in any dish. So no fighting in the kitchen! Keep it a happy place, and the food will shine as a result.

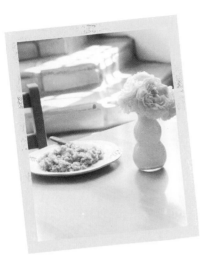

✳ ALWAYS HAVE FRESH FLOWERS OR GREENS ON THE TABLE ✳

Spruce up the table with something simple, such as herbs or greens just picked from outside your home. Try to let this centerpiece reflect the season you are in. Even having a vase pull of plain sticks with a few pine greens in the winter gives a homey touch to the table.

✳ HAVE A CANDLE ON THE TABLE AT ALL TIMES ✳

I prefer natural beeswax candles that produce a soft glow. Lighting a candle is a great way to start a meal; end the meal by blowing it out. This simple act can start to produce a rhythm that the children will appreciate and will make your mealtimes feel special. This one act will help your children will understand that this is an important time of day.

✳ SAY A BLESSING ✳

Honor the food, the farmer, and the cook when you eat. This act of reverence does not have to be religious in nature; just a simple gesture of appreciation for the bounty on your table which will teach your little ones gratitude at an early age.

Here is an example a lovely family meal blessing that we say at our table:

> *Earth who gives to us this food,*
> *Sun who makes it ripe and good,*
> *Farmers we thank you for your work,*
> *Dear Earth, dear sun, dear farmer and cook,*
> *And all those who help us live,*
> *Our loving thanks to you we give.*

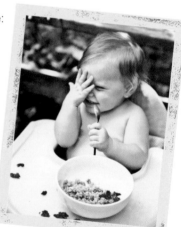

✳ HAVE A SEAT FOR EVERYONE ✳

Make sure everyone, even Baby, has a seat at the table. Rather than seat your baby in a high chair separate from the main table, bring him close enough to feel included in the family meal.

✳ CHOOSE VESSELS WITH CARE ✳

Instead of using plastics for baby, which can be filled with bisphenol A (BPA) toxins, try using wooden bowls or enamelware. I have also found that sippy cups are not needed. Babies can learn early to drink straight from a cup if you take the time to teach them. There will be a few accidents, but that is okay. If you want to use a sippy cup, try the stainless steel sippy cups from Life Without Plastic (which you can get online). These choices make for a beautiful aesthetic table, are better for the environment, and do not allow the food to take on that plastic taste that you sometimes get.

Anni's Quick and Natural Parenting Tips

> Breastfeed your baby as long as possible.
> Eat fresh, organic food that is in season.
> Encourage family rhythms.
> Live simply. Kids do not need so much stuff! Reduce the amount of stuff you give your children and instead encourage them to play with objects they may find in nature or allow them to create games or toys with you as much as possible.
> Kill your television! Kids do not need it, and never allow your baby to watch television. Allow your children's imaginations to grow and prosper without the influence of media.
> Keep your house organized and use natural cleaners. Get rid of any toxic junk—anything containing chemical ingredients that you cannot pronounce should be the first to go!
> Look into homeopathy for natural remedies to common ailments such as colds, flu, sinus problems, or tummy aches.
> No yelling.
> Laugh a lot and use humor whenever you can.
> Offer your children alternatives instead of immediately saying, "no." That word gets old, quick!
> Kiss and hug your kids every chance you get!
> Hold regular family meetings to hear how things are going with each family member.
> Read up on family beds and consider not buying a crib at all.
> Most importantly, remember that your children are little for a very short time. They are kids for about 16 years (before they feel like adults) and adults for about 80 years! Enjoy the time you have with them by listening, honoring, nurturing, and having a ton of fun!

Food Is Best When Made with Love

Feeding your family fresh home-cooked meals is a lot of work and requires a commitment on your part. Remember that it is your love for them that makes this possible. It is the love you put directly in the food that makes it taste better than anyone else's, and it's your love that brings your family together around the table, to share food and create lifelong memories. Give yourself a huge pat on the back and know that this investment you are making now will have a huge effect on your children's culinary experience and nutritional development for the rest of their lives.

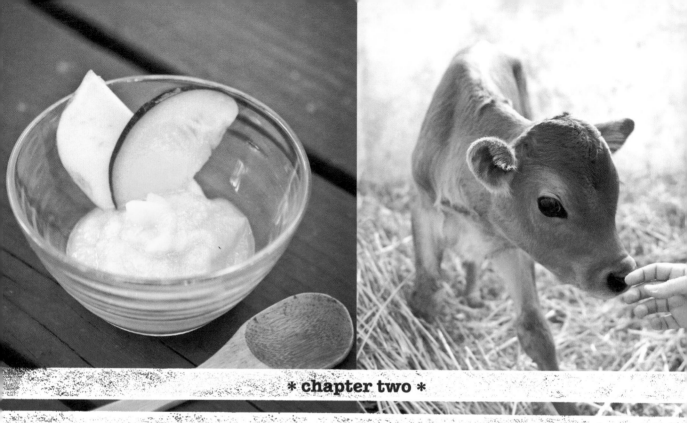

spring purées

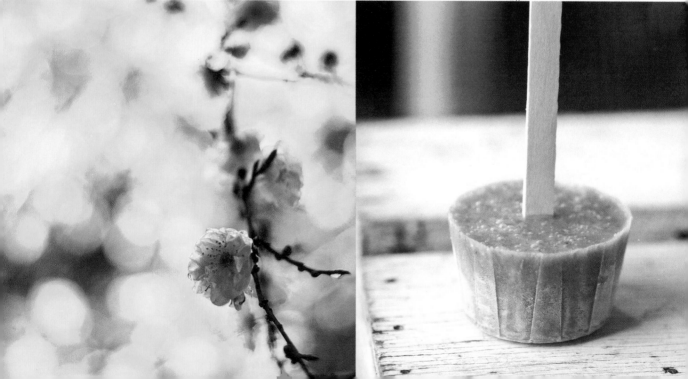

Welcome to spring, where new life blossoms all around, and the chill of winter is passing.

New buds are bursting on the trees, babies are crawling around smelling fresh flowers, kids are starting to get dirty again, and the earth is ready for young seeds. Everyone, and I do mean everyone (Baby included!), wants to eat delicious foods. The problem that many folks have, however, especially those of us with multiple children, is that lack of time and creativity often rule the day when we are rushing around trying to fulfill a million other responsibilities.

I am not going to mislead you by saying cooking for your baby and family takes no time or effort. Cooking in general takes time and effort, but when you take on making fresh homemade baby food, that is an additional task that you must dedicate yourself to. I believe, however, this may be the most important task you can charge yourself with because baby's first foods can shape her culinary palate for a lifetime. This is her fresh start, and you are in the driver's seat of her nutritional health.

I want you to feel confident in the kitchen, and to do that, you may need a few tips and tricks. This book was inspired by my hope that offering you ways to incorporate the baby food into your family meals will allow you to use your precious time in efficient ways that support your goal of feeding your family well, while also teaching your children food traditions that will last a lifetime.

Embracing Growth and New Life

In the spirit of spring, new life, growth, and starting family traditions, it's wonderful to dive into this journey with a fresh perspective on cooking, buying food, and time spent in the kitchen. We spend much of our time rushing, especially in the kitchen, which is why so many folks eat processed, unhealthy fast foods. The trick is changing our perspective in what we value. Time spent in the kitchen does not have to be you working away by yourself over a hot stove. Rather, time spent choosing and growing food, learning from your local farmers and purveyors, prepping and cooking meals, and eventually eating together can be family time. This time spent together teaches your children how to value what they put in their bodies while learning to appreciate the process of where their food comes from and how our choices affect our environment.

Eating fresh, local, seasonal, and organic food is not a pipe dream like some folks may think. It can be a reality for you if you decide to be in charge of your food destiny. Grasping this concept is important because so many of our food choices come from marketing and sales teams around the country who desperately try to persuade us to buy the fast burger or shelf-stable baby food because we don't have the time or skills to make meals at home for our families. This is where shifting what we value comes into play. If we value eating delicious, nutritionally sound foods, then being in the kitchen becomes our joy and not our burden. If we see family meals as a time to

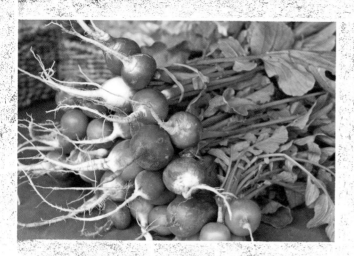
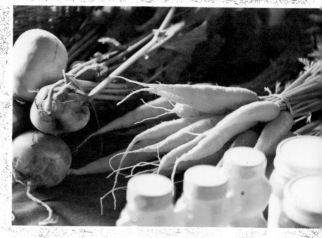

sit together, talk, and enjoy each other's company, rather than just a quick bite to feed the body, then we don't worry about spending too much time in the kitchen and instead focus on passing down food traditions to our children that will benefit their whole lives.

Food is the essence of life, and when we start our babies off on the right track and include our children in the growing, choosing, and cooking, process, we set up foundations that are not easily broken.

Why Fresh?

Have you ever wondered how they make commercially prepared, shelf-stable baby food (the stuff you see on the shelf in your local grocery store)? To kill pathogens and prevent the food from spoiling, the food must be heated to a high temperature. This process kills most of the nutritional value, color, and taste, and the food can sit on the shelf for up to two years! That means the food you buy off the shelf could potentially be older than your baby when you are starting to feed him solids.

Fresh food is superior in every way. Just like us, babies care about what they eat, and fresh food not only just plain tastes better, it is far more nutritious. Giving Baby fresh food allows him to sample what different foods really taste like. Highly processed foods are devoid of flavor and natural texture, so it's hard to distinguish unique tastes. Further, making your own baby food allows you the option to offer your baby far more variety than would ever be available in store bought brands.

Although purées can be frozen, I recommend that babies eat fresh food whenever possible. The shelf life of fresh food if stored in airtight glass jars is seven to ten days refrigerated. Fresh food is far superior to frozen, and frozen foods begin to break down over time. This means the longer they are frozen, the less nutritional value they hold.

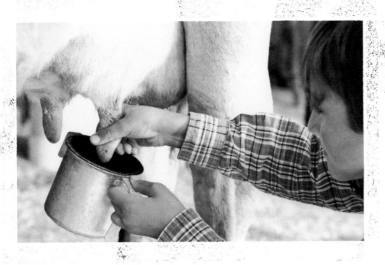
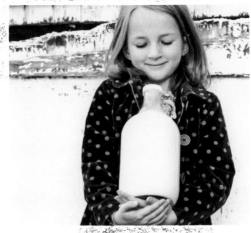

Milk After Age One

After age one, you can start to introduce your baby to other dairy milk while maintaining your breastfeeding routine.

> **Raw Milk:** Raw milk is unpasteurized milk straight from the source. The cow is milked and then you drink it. Where I live in Chester Springs, Pennsylvania, we get the most amazing raw milk, and its creamy flavor is truly unbeatable. We have a local farm that milks the cows and bottles it up for us.
>
> People worry about raw milk, but as long as the cows have not been injected with hormones or antibiotics, are grass fed and allowed to roam freely, raw milk is safe and delicious. If you ever have a chance to get your kids over to a dairy farm to meet cows, and maybe even milk them, they get to see the source of where their milk comes from and learn an appreciation for these amazing animals who give so much of themselves for us.

> **Whole Milk:** If you choose pasteurized milk, make sure it's certified organic. Cow's milk that is not certified organic is typically filled with hormones and antibiotics that were given to the cows who tend to live in very unsanitary living conditions. Choose your dairy wisely and always make it organic (even if you're not an all-organic shopper).

> **Rice Milk:** Made from rice, this is an alternative to cow products. Lactose intolerant folks can have it, and vegans and vegetarians often choose it as a substitute to cow's milk. It has little protein, however, and is often fortified with vitamins. You can also try almond milk for a substitute.

> **Hemp Milk:** Hemp milk is made from hemp seeds and is another healthy alternative to cow's milk. It is great for vegans and vegetarians and is a good source of protein. It has a nutty flavor that many people enjoy.

Blueberry, Raisin, and Almond Purée

8+ months

YIELD: 1½ CUPS (375 G), OR 3 BABY SERVINGS

2-IN-1 OPTION: **OATMEAL PARFAIT WITH TOASTED ALMOND SLIVERS**, PAGE 48

Blueberries are a super antioxidant, raisins are high in iron, and this recipe has the added bonus of almond protein. The alluring bright purple color of this recipe combined with its great taste make this one a winner with most babies right out of the gate.

2 cups (300 g) blueberries
¼ cup (36 g) raisins
1 tablespoon (6 g) ground almonds

1. Wash berries with water and steam with raisins for 3 to 5 minutes, until the berries are soft.
2. Reserve the water from the steamer.
3. Blend the blueberry-raisin mixture in a blender until puréed. Add 1 teaspoon of reserved water at a time, if necessary, until desired consistency is achieved.
4. Add in ground almonds and mix together.
5. Transfer the berry mixture to a bowl and serve warm.

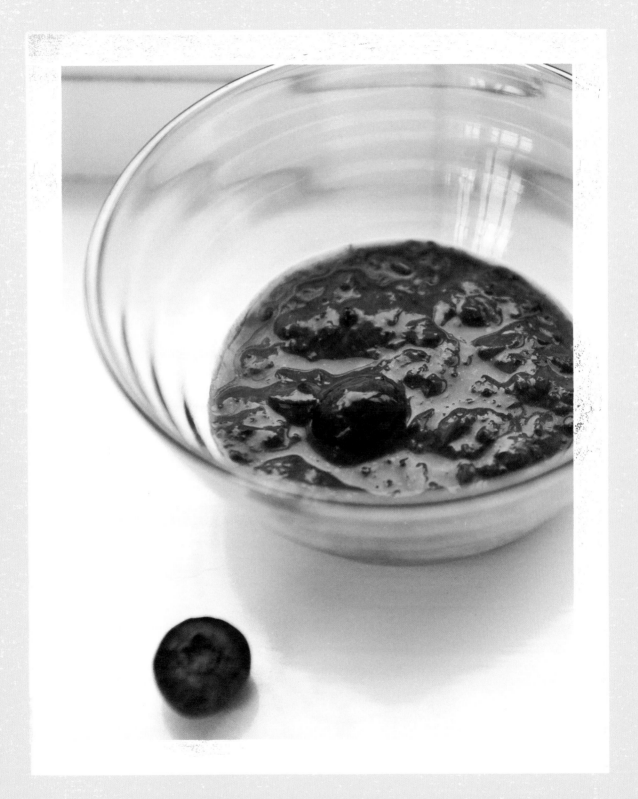

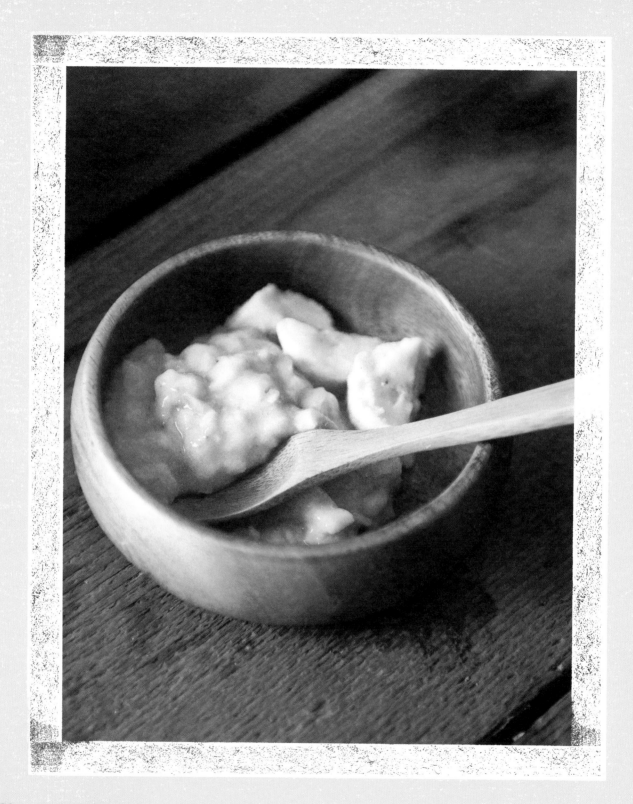

Bountiful Baby Purées

Pure Banana Purée

6+ months

YIELD: 1½ CUPS (375 G), OR 3 BABY SERVINGS

2-IN-1 OPTION: **TROPICAL TILAPIA EN PAPILLOTE,** PAGE 50

Bananas are a great source of dietary fiber and vitamin C. They are naturally sweet and easily digestible, so they are a great first food your baby. Bananas are also a great "on-the-go" baby food because you can mash one up anywhere you go.

2 bananas

1. Peel and crush the banana with a fork, or purée until smooth in a mixer or blender.

The Slow Food Movement

What is the "slow food movement" and why should you care about it? Slow food is sort of the opposite of fast "junk" food and incorporates the fundamental ideologies of community, sustainability, and honoring new and old food traditions. It also supports local farmers and is helping reshape how we see and feel about food in this country. Food is meant to bring people together, nourish our bodies, and connect us to the land and each other. The slow food movement recognizes that many of these traditions have been lost and is trying to bring them back. The movement is especially important for children to learn about because they are our future. We need to pass the shovel to them to continue our growing traditions. If we do not do this responsibly, with our very fragile ecosystem, we risk losing even more precious natural resources and disempowering our children to take on these responsibilities with pride and awareness.

Plum and Fuji Apple Purée

6+ months

YIELD: 1½ CUPS (375 G), OR 4 BABY SERVINGS

2-IN-1 OPTION: **PLUM TART WITH BRIE AND HONEY-ROASTED WALNUTS,** PAGE 51

....

Yum! This sweet dynamic duo is a crowd pleaser. It's the perfect combination of tart and sweet and is a nice starter baby food. It's easy on the tummy and keeps babies wanting more. My daughter loved this combination, and I must admit that I too took a few bites here and there.

2 plums, peeled and cubed
2 Fuji apples, peeled and cubed

1. Steam plums and apples together for 7 to 9 minutes, until they are soft.
2. Reserve the water from the steamer.
3. Blend the plum-apple mixture in a blender until puréed. Add 1 teaspoon (5 ml) of reserved water at a time, if necessary, until desired consistency is achieved.

spring purées

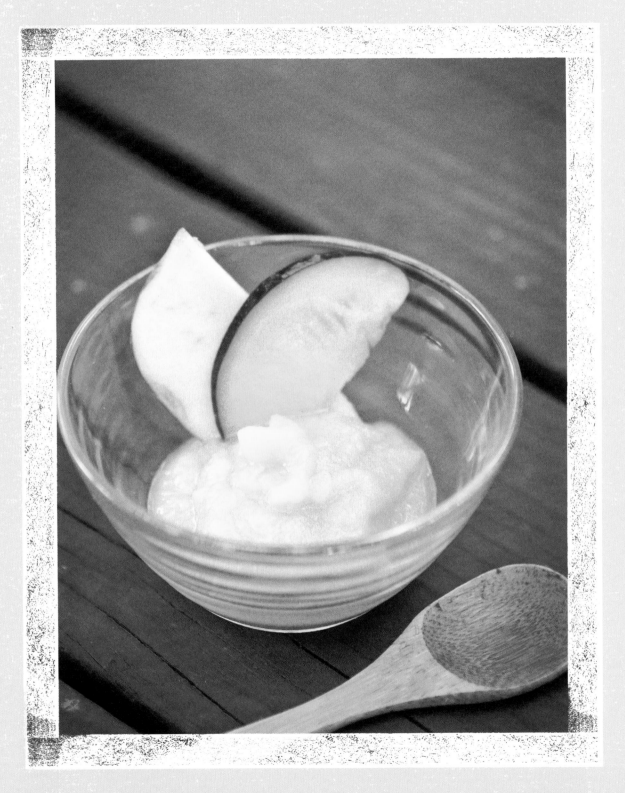

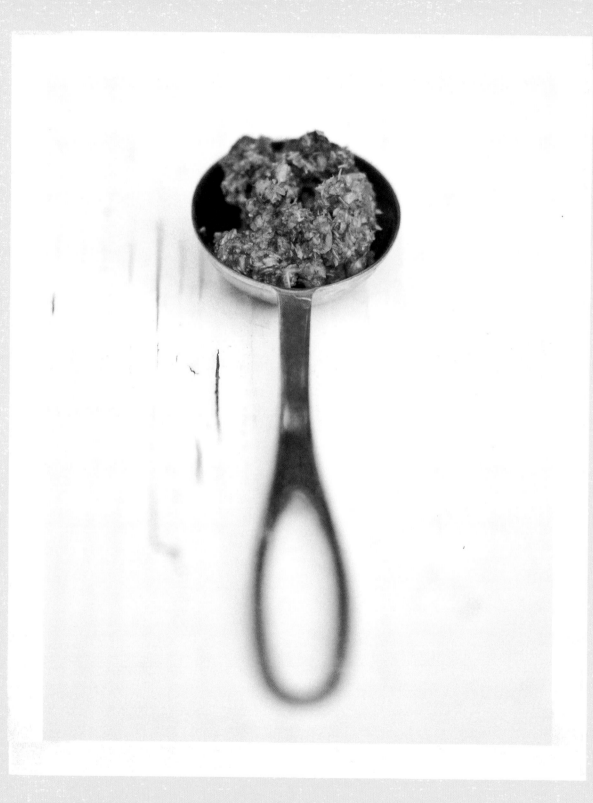

Bountiful Baby Purées

Spinach, Kale, and Banana Purée

7+ months

YIELD: 2 CUPS (500 G), OR 4 BABY SERVINGS

2-IN-1 OPTION: **VEGGIE TORTILLA CHEESE MELTS,** PAGE 52

This is a super-high nutritionally valued meal, and the added sweet kick of the banana makes this a pleasing bite for any baby. Spinach and kale are super foods and contain protein and iron. Getting your kids hooked on greens is the way to go, so try this one at least once a week. I still turn this purée into ice pops for my older kids.

1 cup (30 g) spinach leaves, packed
1 cup (30 g) kale leaves, chopped and packed, stems removed
2 bananas, peeled and sliced

1. Steam spinach and kale together for 3 minutes, until they are soft.
2. Reserve the water from the steamer.
3. Blend the spinach and kale mixture in a blender with the banana slices until puréed. Add 1 teaspoon (5 ml) of reserved water at a time, if necessary, until desired consistency is achieved.

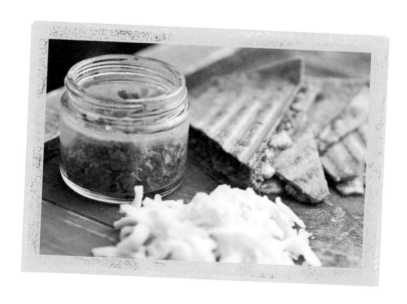

Mushroom, Onion, Broccoli and Herb Textured Purée

11+ months

YIELD: 2 CUPS (500 G), OR 4 BABY SERVINGS

2-IN-1 OPTION: **CREAMY SPRING QUICHE**, PAGE 53

....

This is a savory dish that is meant for your baby when he is a little more advanced in his eating skills. The flavors are irresistible, and using high quality products is the key to this meal—use mushrooms from your local farmers' market if possible. Onions are the most under-valued vegetable, but they are like the best friend to which you turn to make everything better. Giving your young children a healthy appreciation of the onion is so important because it's the base flavor in so many meals. I always say as long as I have an onion in the house, I can make anything taste good.

1 tablespoon (15 g) coconut oil
1 cup (70 g) good quality shiitake mushrooms, chopped small
1 yellow onion, chopped
1 cup (70 g) of broccoli florets, chopped small
1 teaspoon oregano
1 teaspoon thyme
1 tablespoon (15 ml) Bragg Liquid Aminos

1. In a sauté pan, heat coconut on high heat. Once the oil is hot, turn heat to medium.
2. Add in the mushrooms, onion, and broccoli and sauté approximately 6 to 7 minutes until lightly browned.
3. Add in the herbs and liquid aminos and sauté until softened.
4. Put mixture in blender and pulse for a moment to get the food a little less chunky. You want this dish to be textured, not completely smooth.
5. Serve warm.

RECIPE NOTES
....

❯ If you plan on using this recipe for the *Creamy Spring Quiche*, set 1½ cups (365 g) aside before pulsing in the blender.
❯ Bragg Liquid Aminos is a natural liquid protein concentrate, derived from soybeans. It contains important healthy amino acids and protein and is a great addition to veggies, grains, meat dishes, and more.

Pure English Peas Purée

6+ months

YIELD: 1½ CUPS (375 ML), OR 4 BABY SERVINGS

2-IN-1 OPTION: **FRESH PEA SOUP WITH BASIL BUTTER,** PAGE 54

There are nothing like sweet fresh English peas, especially if they are straight from your baby food garden. I know this is somewhat labor intensive, but the difference in taste is incredible. English peas are expensive, so I do suggest throwing them in your garden plot, and when they are ready, your older children can help pick and shell, which is fun and appetizing.

1 pound (455 g) fresh English peas, shelled

1. Steam peas for 4 to 5 minutes, until they are soft.
2. Reserve the water from the steamer.
3. Blend the peas in a blender until puréed. Add 1 teaspoon (5 ml) of reserved water at a time, if necessary, until desired consistency is achieved.

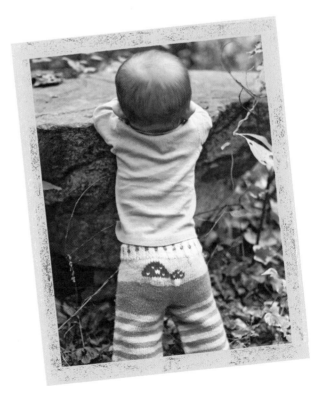

Spinach, Pineapple, and Plain Yogurt Purée

7+ months

YIELD: 3 CUPS (750 G), OR 8 TO 10 BABY SERVINGS

2-IN-1 OPTION: **GREEN GOODNESS ICE POPS,** PAGE 55

....

Spinach is power packed with protein, antioxidants, and essential vitamins. It loses its nutritional punch after about a week after being picked, so this is a great veggie to grow yourself or source from your local community-supported agriculture (CSA) group or farmer's market. No need to steam this recipe, just pop in all in the blender and hit the purée button.

1½ cups (45 g) spinach leaves, packed

1 whole pineapple, outside cut off and chopped into chunks

1½ cups (345 g) plain yogurt

1. Blend the spinach, pineapple, and yogurt together in a blender until desired consistency is achieved.

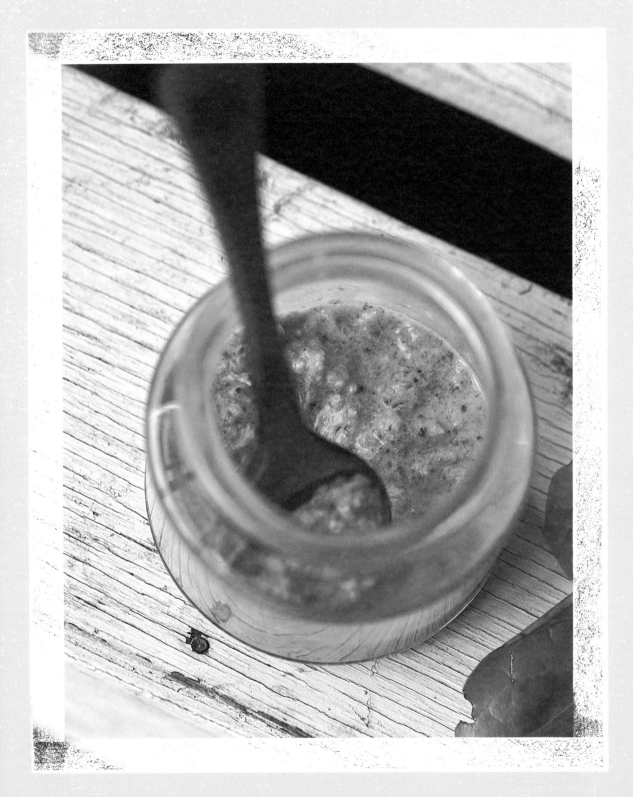

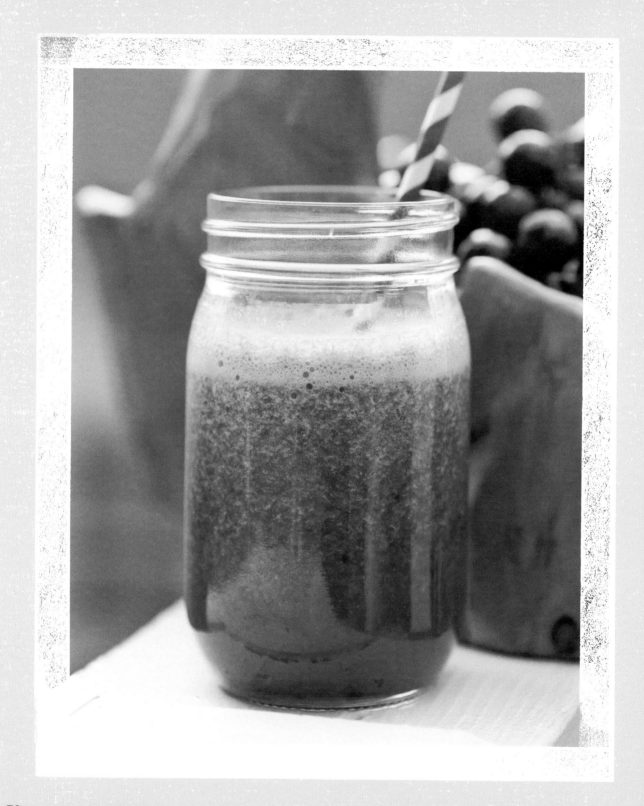

Cherry, Kiwi, and Pineapple Smoothie

10+ months

YIELD: 3 CUPS (750 G), OR 6 BABY SERVINGS

2-IN-1 OPTION: **SPRING GARDEN SALAD WITH GRAPES AND SWEET CHERRY VINAIGRETTE,** PAGE 56

....

I could drink truckloads of this smoothie. I guarantee you and your baby will love it. This is a great first try at drinking a little something in a cup. Make sure you only offer little sips and add as much water as you need to get it to a smooth drinking consistency that suits your baby. Cherries are packed with antioxidants, and when they come in season in your region, eat as many as you can. They are truly a treat from nature and offer many health benefits that will boost your immunity.

**2 cups (300 g) fresh Bing cherries,
    pitted or fresh frozen organic cherries**

2 kiwis, peeled and sliced

1 whole pineapple, skins cut off and cubed

½ cup (120 ml) of water

½ cup (150 g) ice

1. Blend all ingredients in a blender until puréed into a chilled smoothie.

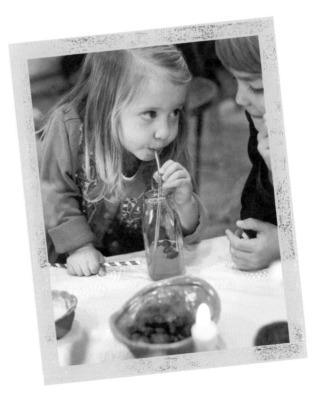

Apricot, Raisins, Carrot, Flax, and Walnut Purée

9+ months

YIELD: 1½ CUPS (375 G) OR 3 BABY SERVINGS

2-IN-1 OPTION: **FRUIT AND NUT STICKY BUNS,** PAGE 57

This tart and nutty purée will bring a smile to your baby's face. The walnuts add protein, and the apricots give this healthy combo a boost of vitamin C.

1 cup fresh (165 g) or dried (130 g) apricots
¼ cup (36 g) raisins
1 carrot, sliced
1 tablespoon (12 g) flaxseed
1 tablespoon (5 g) ground walnuts
    (Use a coffee grinder for quick and easy grinding results.)

1. Allow apricots, raisins, and carrot to steam together for approximately 9 minutes, or until they are all soft.
2. Reserve the water from the steamer.
3. Blend the mixture in a blender until puréed. Add 1 teaspoon (5 ml) of reserved water at a time, if necessary, until desired consistency is achieved.
4. Add in ground walnuts and mix together.
5. Transfer the apricot mixture to a bowl and serve warm.

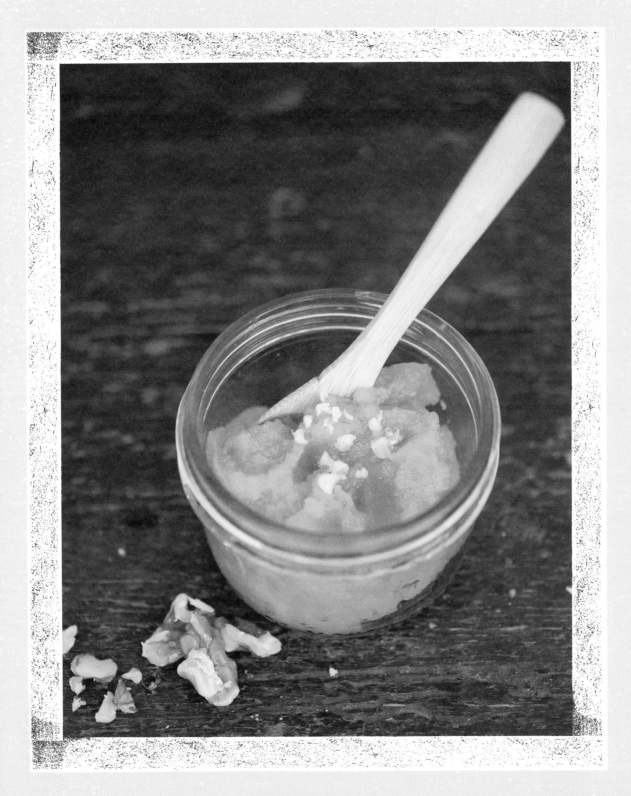

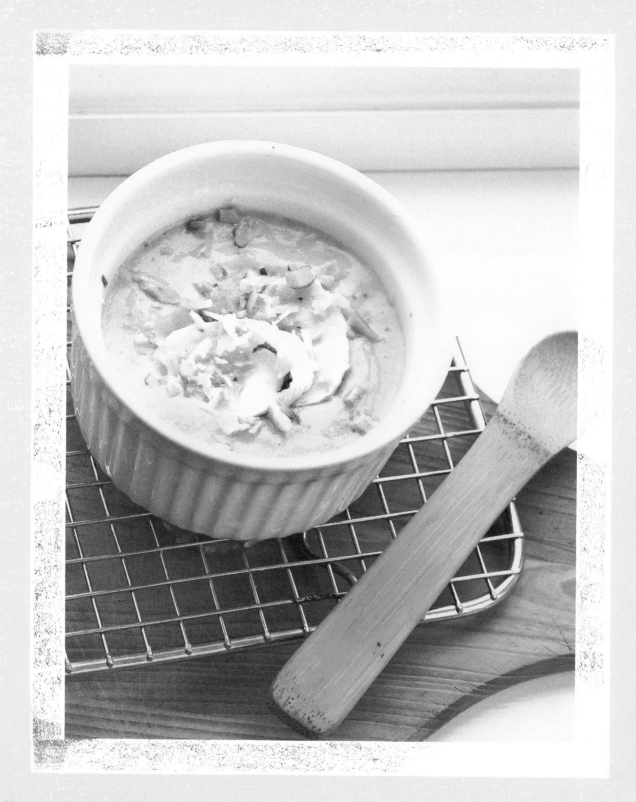

Banana, Almond Butter, and Flax Purée

9+ months

YIELD: 2 CUPS (500 G), OR 4 BABY SERVINGS

2-IN-1 OPTION: **BREAKFAST ICE POPS,** PAGE 58

This is a fun way to give your baby protein. Almond butter is super easy to make from scratch as well, if you are motivated. Just grind almonds in a food processor until they turn into a paste and then eventually almond butter. That is it! My 4-year-old likes to spread this purée onto his crackers for an after school snack.

3 bananas, peeled and sliced
½ cup (130 g) almond butter
1 cup (230 g) of plain organic yogurt
1 tablespoon (8 g) ground flaxseed

1. Blend the bananas, almond butter, yogurt, and flaxseed together in a blender until desired consistency is achieved.

Asparagus and Olive Textured Purée

11+ months

YIELD: 1½ CUPS (375 G), OR 3 BABY SERVINGS

2-IN-1 OPTION: **ASPARAGUS MINI TARTS,** PAGE 59

Asparagus is an amazing vegetable that some folks think is too fancy or too hard to prepare or see them as a delicacy. However, this hearty vegetable is not pretentious at all and offers a hearty boost of vitamins K, C, and A to any child's menu. My kids love to just "grab and go" with these green gems. Sometimes I just give them a quick steam, hit them with some butter and Bragg Liquid Aminos and voila: a great after school snack. For babies, try this combination with the added touch of olive medley to give it just the right flavor.

1 cup (100 g) fresh asparagus, chopped
¼ cup (50 g) variety of olives, minced
1 garlic clove, minced
¼ teaspoon Bragg Liquid Aminos

1. Steam asparagus for approximately 7 minutes, or until they are all softened but still firm.
2. Reserve the water from the steamer.
3. In a blender, add the asparagus, olive medley, garlic, and liquid aminos and blend until desired textured is achieved. I think this meal is best served with a little texture and is meant for an older baby who can already chew and has been eating for at least two months.
4. Transfer the asparagus mixture to a bowl and serve warm.

Kale, Banana, and Hemp Seed Purée

7+ months

YIELD: 2 CUPS (500 G), OR 4 BABY SERVINGS

2-IN-1 OPTION: **SWEET GREEN QUINOA,** PAGE 59

Kale is one of the healthiest foods around, super high in antioxidants, and, when combined with yummy bananas and protein-packed hemp seed, it makes for a winning baby purée. Hemp seed has the most essential fatty and amino acids of any plant resource and is the most easily digestible. It is becoming mainstream and easily accessible. You should be able to buy it at your local health food grocer or online. Try sprinkling a little ground hemp seed on a warm whole grain breakfast cereal for baby and you.

2 cups (60 g) kale

1 banana

¼ cup (35 g) hemp seeds, ground in coffee grinder

1. Wash the kale and cut into pieces.
2. Steam the kale for 5 to 7 minutes, or until soft. Reserve the liquid from the steamer.
3. Transfer the kale to a food processor.
4. Add in banana, ¼ cup (60 ml) of the reserved liquid, and ground hemp seeds.
5. Purée until smooth. Continue to add the reserved liquid in scant 2 tablespoons (28 ml) increments until the purée is to desired consistency.

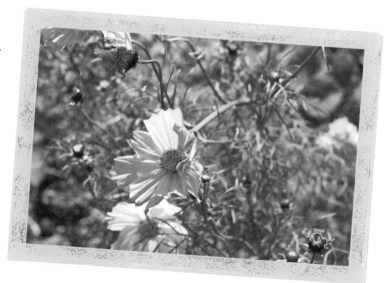

Millet and Cheddar Purée

11+ months

YIELD: 1½ CUPS (375 G), OR 4 BABY SERVINGS

2-IN-1 OPTION: **FUN CHEDDAR CRISP CRACKERS,** PAGE 60

Millet is an amazingly easy grain for babies to digest, and other flavors marry well with this versatile protein. The trick is using a coffee grinder or small blender, to grind down the millet to a powder, which makes it easy to make a little baby meal. Try substituting the cheddar for a fruit or vegetable purée and adding it to the millet if your baby is younger.

1½ cups (350 ml) water
½ cup (60 g) millet, ground down to a powder
½ cup (58 g) shredded sharp Cheddar cheese

1. Bring water to a boil, add the millet, and turn down to a simmer, stirring frequently for about 10 minutes.

2. As the millet starts forming into a cereal-type consistency, add the cheese.

3. Let the cheese melt into the mixture.

4. Serve warm.

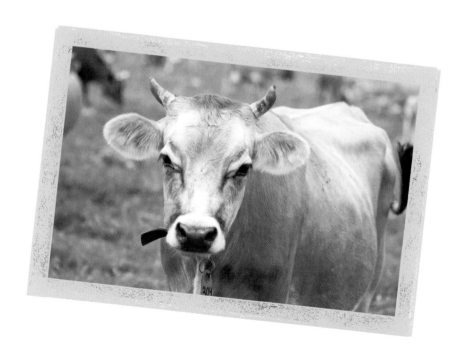

Roasted Eggplant Purée

9+ months

YIELD: 1½ CUPS (375 G), OR 4 BABY SERVINGS

2-IN-1 OPTION: **EGGPLANT SALSA,** PAGE 60

....

Eggplant is a delicious delicacy to introduce to your baby. The nutty flavor is unique and offers him a nice boost of vitamin C and potassium. Eggplant is a great meat alternative for vegetarians as well, as it can be made into a fantastic veggie burger with its meaty texture.

2 purple globe eggplants, cut down the middle
1 tablespoon (15 ml) olive oil

1. Preheat the oven to 350° F (180° C, or gas mark 4).
2. Oil the eggplants and roast for 15 to 20 minutes.
3. Allow to cool and peel off the skin.
4. Place the eggplant in the blender and purée to desired consistency.

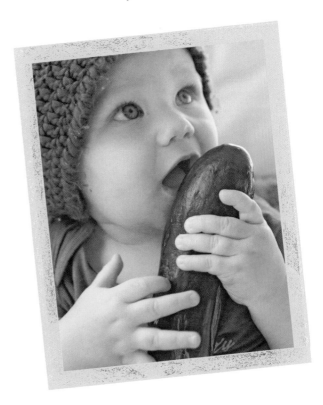

Parmesan Potato Purée

11+ months

YIELD: 3 CUPS (750 G), OR 6 BABY SERVINGS

2-IN-1 OPTION: **PARMESAN CRUSTED HALIBUT WITH LEMON-CAPER SAUCE,** PAGE 61

Who doesn't love cheesy potatoes? Babies especially like this creamy version. Coconut milk is rich in omega-3 fatty acid, fiber, and protein and is a great drink for your toddlers. If you can't find yellow Finn potatoes, which have a very creamy, buttery flavor, substitute Yukon Gold.

6 yellow Finn potatoes, peeled and cubed
½ cup (50 g) freshly grated Parmesan cheese
¼ cup (60 ml) coconut milk
Dash of pepper

1. Place potatoes in a medium sized pot of water and bring to a boil.
2. Boil potatoes until soft, about 12 minutes.
3. Drain water from the pot and transfer to a blender.
4. Blend the potatoes with cheese, coconut milk, and pepper.
5. Serve warm.

Save that Veggie Bath Water!

It is important to reserve the water from steaming fruits and vegetables. Nutrients from the food leech into the water, and you want to add those nutrients back into your purée. If you have leftover water from steaming fruit, add it to some tea for a flavorful twist. Leftover water from steaming veggies can be added to soups or for boiling rice and other grains.

Apricot Raspberry Purée

8+ months

YIELD: 1½ CUPS (375 G), OR 4 BABY SERVINGS

2-IN-1 OPTION: **APRICOT AND RASPBERRY FRUIT LEATHER,** PAGE 61

Yum! This is a super-sweet and inviting purée to make for your little sweetie. It's also a great purée to turn into jam, salad dressing, or breakfast yogurt I love this combination, and as simple as it is, the flavors are just perfect together. I guarantee success with this one!

4 apricots, diced
1½ cups (200 g) raspberries

1. Steam apricots for about 5 minutes. Add the raspberries and steam for an additional 2 minutes.
2. Reserve the water from the steamer.
3. Blend the apricot–raspberry mixture in a blender until puréed. Add 1 teaspoon (5 ml) of reserved water at a time, if necessary, until desired consistency is achieved.

Oatmeal Parfait with Toasted Almond Slivers

15+ months

YIELD: 4 CUPS (1 KG), OR 2 ADULT SERVINGS OR 4 KID SERVINGS

Steel-cut oats are a wonderful breakfast for anyone in your family. One cup has 8 grams of fiber. Having a warm breakfast in the morning is satisfying, and turning this dish into a little parfait is fun for the kids and a unique spin on a morning classic.

1 cup (80 g) steel-cut oats
3 cups (700 ml) water
1 cup (235 ml) of raw milk or whole milk
1 tablespoon (14 g) unsalted butter
1 tablespoon (20 g) honey
2 tablespoons (30 g) *Blueberry, Raisin, and Almond Purée*, page 24
2 tablespoons (14 g) almond slivers, toasted (optional)
¼ cup (38 g) fresh blueberries for topping

1. Place slivered almonds in a sauté pan on medium heat (dry, no oil required). Toast for about 5 minutes and set aside. If your baby does not chew yet, please do not include the almonds.

2. In a large saucepan, bring water to a boil.

3. Add steel-cut oats and stir occasionally for 20 to 25 minutes until soft.

4. Add milk, butter, and honey.

5. Add *Blueberry, Raisin, and Almond Purée* and mix.

6. In glass jar or cup, create a parfait by adding a layer of the cooked oatmeal, followed by a layer of the puree. Top with toasted almonds and fresh blueberries.

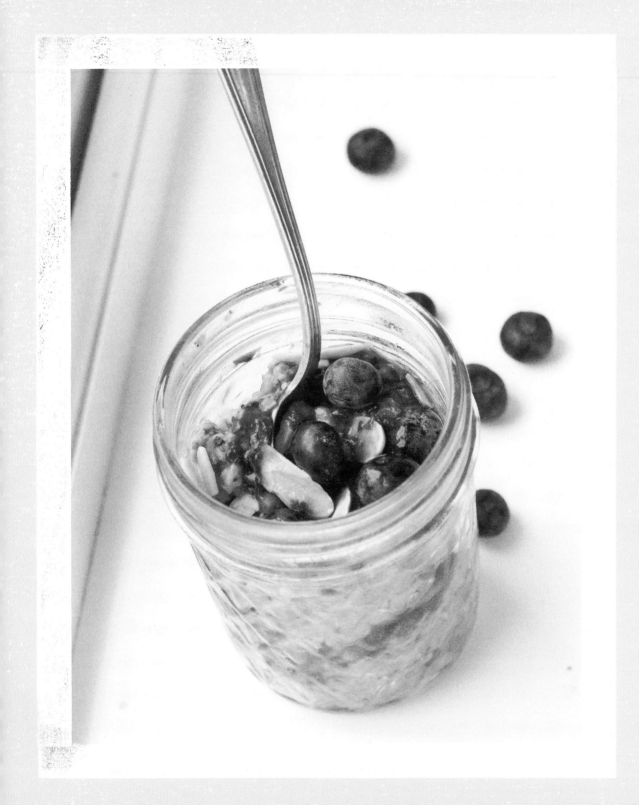

Tropical Tilapia en Papillote

15+ months

YIELD: 3 ADULT SERVINGS OR 6 KID SERVINGS

Tilapia is a mild flavored fish that takes well to a variety of flavor profiles. Adding the banana purée to this fish dish gives it a tropical flavor. You may even consider serving black beans and mango salsa on the side. It's fun to serve your guests their fish in the cooked parchment paper (*en papillote*), as it makes a pleasing aesthetic for your meal.

3 fillets of fresh wild-caught tilapia
¼ teaspoon each of salt and pepper per fillet
3 tablespoons *Pure Banana Purée* (page 27), divided
1 tablespoon (14 g) unsalted butter, divided
9 sprigs fresh thyme, divided
1 tablespoon capers (10 g), divided
2 garlic cloves, minced and divided

1. Preheat oven to 350°F (180°C, or gas mark 4).
2. Tear three sheets of parchment baking paper into large enough squares to completely wrap each piece of fish.
3. Place each fillet onto a piece of parchment paper.
4. Sprinkle each fillet with salt and pepper and top with *Pure Banana Purée*.
5. Top each piece of fish with butter, 3 sprigs of fresh thyme, capers, and garlic.
6. Fold up the corners of the parchment so that a tent forms over each fillet.
7. Place wrapped fish in a shallow baking dish and place in the oven.
8. Bake for 12 to 15 minutes.
9. Serve warm in paper wrappings.

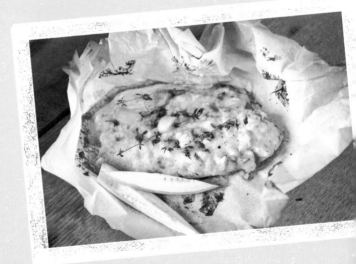

Plum Tart with Brie and Honey-Roasted Walnuts

18+ months

YIELD: 8 TO 10 TARTS, OR SERVINGS

Oh my goodness, this is good! This tart is the perfect combination of sweet and savory, and it looks super fancy. I love desserts that look like it took me several days to make, but actually only took 15 minutes. If you decide to go the extra mile and top it with a little freshly whipped cream, you will likely having your family begging for seconds and thirds! Note that you will need a mandolin slicer for this recipe.

FOR TOPPING:
½ cup (120 g) chopped walnuts
¼ cup (85 g) honey for walnuts

FOR TART:
1 sheet puff pastry, chilled, not frozen
1 cup (245 g) *Plum and Fuji Apple Purée*, page 28
½ cup (75 g) cubed Brie cheese
1 plum, sliced thin with a mandolin slicer
¼ cup (85 g) honey for drizzling

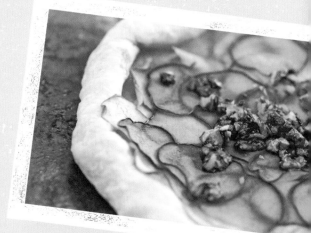

1. Preheat oven to 350°F (180°C, or gas mark 4). Line a cookie sheet with parchment paper.
2. In a small saucepan on medium heat, combine the walnuts and ¼ cup of honey. Stir to coat the walnuts.
3. Pour the honey-coated walnuts onto the lined baking sheet and cook for about 10 minutes. Set aside.
4. Roll out puff pastry on a floured surface into a rustic, imperfect circle, about ¼-inch (6 mm)-thick. Create an edge on all sides by rolling up some pastry. Poke a fork in the center of the dough a couple of times. Move the dough to its own parchment-lined cookie sheet.
5. Spread the *Plum and Fuji Apple Purée* on top of the puff pastry.
6. Add chunks of Brie cheese on top of the purée mixture.
7. Top with sliced plums, honey, and the walnut topping.
8. Bake on the prepared cookie sheet for 15 to 18 minutes, until pastry has puffed up and is golden brown in color.
9. Serve warm.

Veggie Tortilla Cheese Melts

18+ months

YIELD: 2 ADULT SERVINGS OR 4 KID SERVINGS

....

All kids love cheesy melted foods, and this version kicks up the healthy with the added veggie purée. The purée also gives this dish a depth of flavor that adults will love. I know the banana might not sound like it would taste good, but it works!

4 veggie tortillas, any variety and size you like
1 cup (245 g) *Spinach, Kale, and Banana Purée* (page 31), divided
1 cup (80 g) Havarti cheese, shredded and divided
1 teaspoon coconut oil for cooking pan

1. Lay out a tortilla and top it with one-half of the *Spinach, Kale, and Banana Purée* and one-half of the cheese. Cover prepared tortilla with another tortilla.

2. Repeat for the other two remaining tortillas.

3. In a sauté pan on medium heat, heat coconut oil until hot. Place one fully assembled tortilla "sandwich" in the pan.

4. After about 3 minutes, flip the whole thing.

5. Let each side get a little crispy and allow the cheese to melt.

6. Repeat with the other tortilla "sandwiches."

7. Cut into triangles for easy eating and serve warm while the cheese is melted.

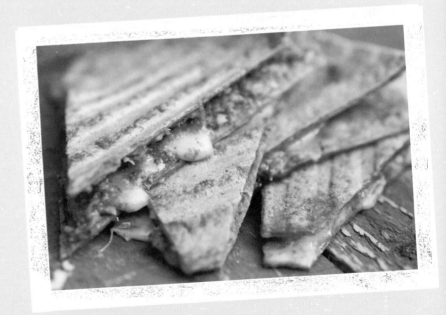

Creamy Spring Quiche

18+ months

YIELD: 6 ADULT SERVINGS, OR 8 KID SERVINGS

Eggs are a perfect way to introduce proteins into your family meals, and a spring quiche is tasty and healthy. This is so easy to prepare and a great warm breakfast to give the day a jump start.

1 teaspoon unsalted butter

2 garlic cloves, minced very small

1½ cups (365 g) *Mushroom, Onion, Broccoli, and Herb Textured Purée* (page 32), before pulsing it in your blender, if possible

1 cup (115 g) shredded cheddar cheese

½ cup (115 g) cream cheese

6 eggs

½ cup (120 ml) raw milk or whole milk

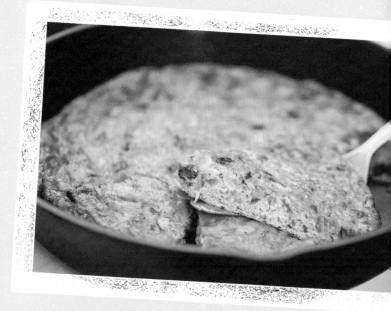

1. Preheat oven to 350°F (180°C, or gas mark 4).

2. In a large saucepan, melt butter over medium heat and add the garlic to start browning. After a few minutes, add *mushroom, onion, broccoli, and herb* combination, mix, and set aside.

3. In a large mixing bowl, mix together eggs, milk, and cheese. Add the *mushroom, onion, broccoli, and herb* combination and stir to combine. Ladle egg mixture into a buttered pie dish or cast iron skillet and bake for 40 to 45 minutes or until browned on top.

Fresh Pea Soup with Basil Butter

11+ months

YIELD: 12 CUPS, OR 6 ADULT SERVINGS, OR 10 KID SERVINGS

....

You may wonder if you can substitute freshly shelled peas with store-bought frozen peas, but freshly shelled peas are infinitely tastier. Only make this soup when you have time and a lot of love and little hands around to help. It's just not worth it otherwise. When you make this soup with freshly shelled peas, you can taste the garden, so to speak. The basil butter is a decadent topping that just works with this recipe in a way that is soothing and creamy. It brings all these flavors home. If you want to really impress someone with your cooking or say "I love you" in a big way, make this soup!

FOR THE SOUP:
2 tablespoons (28 g) unsalted butter
1 large yellow onion, chopped
1 large leek, chopped (use the whole thing)
2 garlic cloves, minced
2 teaspoons (12 g) sea salt
2 teaspoons (4 g) pepper
4 cups (1 L) chicken stock
2 cups (500 g) *Pure English Peas Purée*, page 33
3 cups (450 g) freshly shelled peas
1 dash of cayenne pepper
1 chicken bouillon cube

FOR THE BUTTER:
16 fresh chopped basil leaves
3 garlic cloves
1 stick (½ cup, or 112 g) butter
Sea salt and pepper to taste

1. In a large soup pot, melt the butter and sauté the chopped onion, leek, and garlic until browned. Season with salt and pepper.

2. Add the chicken stock, *Pure English Peas Purée*, and the freshly shelled peas. Mix well.

3. Add the cayenne and bouillon to the pot.

4. Using a hand mixer or blender, purée until soup is a smooth consistency.

5. Let simmer to meld the flavors together while you prepare the basil butter.

6. To make the basil butter: Put all the ingredients in a food processor and pulse until well blended.

7. Spoon soup into bowls and top with butter.

Green Goodness Ice Pops

11+ months

YIELD: MAKES ABOUT 20 TO 25 SMALL ICE POPS, OR SERVINGS

....

Turning *Spinach, Pineapple, and Plain Yogurt Purée* into an ice pop is a great way to keep this powerhouse of a purée alive and well in your home, especially if your baby has older siblings. My kids love ice pops and this is one of their favorites. I offer this treat at kids' birthday parties as well, and parents are always happy to hear what is in it. They can hardly believe that their children are gobbling them down.

3 cups (750 g) *Spinach, Pineapple,
   and Plain Yogurt Purée*, page 34
2 bananas, peeled and sliced
1 tablespoon (12 g) whole flaxseed

1. Combine the *Spinach, Pineapple, and Plain Yogurt Purée* with bananas and flaxseed and purée in a blender.

2. Freeze in individual small paper cups with wooden craft sticks or an ice pop mold.

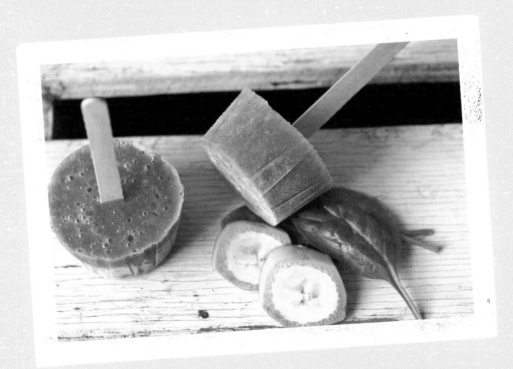

Spring Garden Salad with Grapes and Sweet Cherry Vinaigrette

18+ months

YIELD: 4 ADULT SERVINGS

I love a fresh salad with spring greens, fruit, and veggies. Even if you think your little ones do not like salad, give it a try. I think parents often forget to offer their little kids foods that they perceive as adult foods, and the kids do not even get the opportunity to form an opinion. This simple salad is sweet and savory and has a delicious dressing made with your baby smoothie.

FOR THE SALAD:
3 salad bowls of spring greens
1 zucchini, sliced
1 cup (150 g) grapes, cut in half after measuring
¼ cup (40 g) chopped red onion

FOR THE VINAIGRETTE:
¼ cup (60 g) *Cherry, Kiwi, and Pineapple Smoothie*, page 37
1 shallot, chopped small
1 clove garlic, peeled and chopped
1 tablespoon (20 g) honey
1 tablespoon (11 g) Dijon mustard
2 tablespoons (10 ml) orange juice
¼ cup (60 ml) olive oil
Salt and pepper to taste

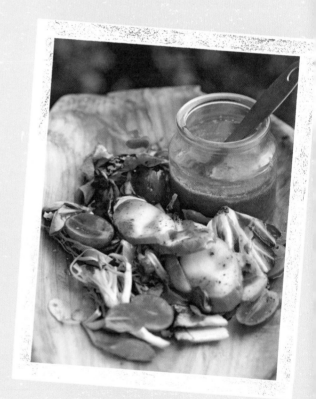

1. Mix greens, zucchini, grapes and red onions together in a large bowl.

2. In a blender, blend *Cherry, Kiwi, and Pineapple Smoothie*, shallot, garlic, honey, mustard, orange juice, salt, and pepper.

3. Slowly stream in the olive oil until well mixed.

4. Drizzle the vinaigrette over the salad and serve warm.

Fruit and Nut Sticky Buns

19+ months

YIELD: 8 TO 10 BUNS, OR SERVINGS

Sticky buns are a treat and everyone knows it. They are decadent and delicious, but when you add in our special complimentary purée, it gives them a healthier twist while still being delicious. These are my weakness, so I am glad I found a way to bring a little nutritional value to my sticky bun recipe.

Al- purpose flour for dusting the work space

1 sheet puff pastry, chilled, not frozen

1 cup (250 g) *Apricot, Raisins, Carrot, Flax, and Walnut Purée*, page 38

1 tablespoon (7 g) cinnamon

2 tablespoons (28 g) unsalted butter, divided melted and softened

¼ cup (85 g) honey, divided

¼ cup (60 g) brown sugar

½ cup (60 g) chopped walnuts

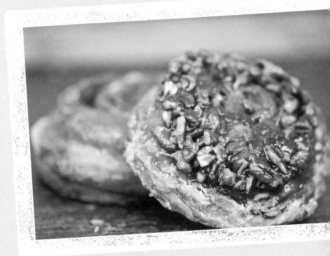

1. Preheat oven to 350°F (180°C, or gas mark 4).

2. In a large bowl, mix together the *Apricot, Raisins, Carrot, Flax, Walnut Purée* with the butter, cinnamon, honey (reserve just a small amount for a light drizzle at the end), and brown sugar.

3. Roll out puff pastry on a floured surface into a rectangle, 12 x 24 inches (30 x 61 cm) and ¼-inch (6 mm)-thick. Melt a little butter and brush over the pastry.

4. Spread the mixture over the dough and roll up like a jelly roll. Pinch seams together with water and flip over to top-side of roll. Cut into slices approximately 1½-inches (4 cm)-thick.

5. Place cut sticky buns, close together or touching each other, in a buttered round 10-inch (25 cm) baking pan or pie pan.

6. Top with chopped walnuts and lightly drizzle a tad more honey.

7. Bake for 15 to 18 minutes until golden brown on top.

8. Serve warm.

Breakfast Ice Pops

11+ months

YIELD: 12 ICE POPS

· ·

Ice pops for breakfast, say what? That's right! These are a quick and healthy bite in the morning. Mom, Dad, and kids can partake of these little gems, which is why I love making them.

2 cups (500 g) *Banana, Almond Butter, and Flax Purée*, page 41
¼ cup (30 g) finely chopped walnuts

1. Combine the *Banana, Almond Butter, and Flax Purée* with chopped walnuts.
2. Freeze in individual paper cups with wooden craft sticks or in an ice pop mold.

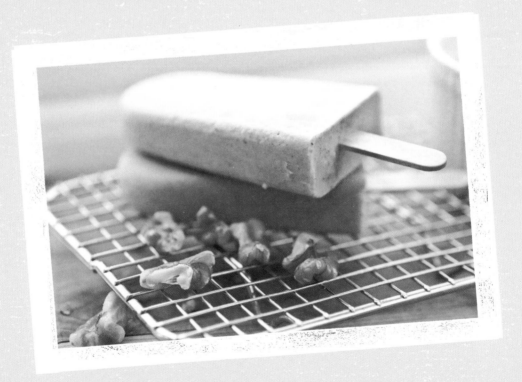

Asparagus Mini Tarts

19+ months

YIELD: 12 TARTS, OR SERVINGS

....

These tarts are fun for kids because they are bite-sized, tasty, and easy to prepare. The kids can help make them. I am all about appetizers for kids, and I love that my friend Rachel sometimes does appetizers for dinner for her two cuties. I think it's brilliant to make a bunch of little appetizers and call it kids tapas night!

All-purpose flour for dusting the work space
1 sheet puff pastry, chilled, not frozen
1 cup (250 g) *Asparagus and Olive Textured Purée*, page 42
½ cup (40 g) shredded Havarti cheese
½ cup (40 g) shredded Parmesan cheese

1. Preheat oven to 350°F (180°C, or gas mark 4).

2. Roll out puff pastry on a floured surface into a rectangle, about 12 x 24 inches (30 x 60 cm) and ¼-inch (6 mm)-thick.

3. Using a 3-inch (7 cm)-round cookie cutter, cut out rounds of puff pastry.

4. Spray a muffin tin with non-stick spray. Place a single round in each of the muffin holes. Using a fork, poke a few holes in the bottom of each pastry round.

5. Scoop about 1 tablespoon (15 g) of the *Asparagus and Olive Textured Purée* mixture into each of the puff pastry rounds and top each with a small amount of cheese.

6. Bake for 10 to 12 minutes until golden brown on top.

7. Serve warm.

Sweet Green Quinoa

11+ months

YIELD: 2 CUPS (490 G) OR 4 SERVINGS

....

Quinoa is a super grain that is packed full of protein. It's great as an alternative to meat, and its nutty flavor is a hit with most toddlers. Combined with *Kale, Banana, and Hemp Seed Purée*, it makes for a super-duper healthy meal—my son Bodhi gobbles it up. This grain is versatile and can be used in both sweet and savory meals. If you have enough leftover purée, add in one additional banana, freeze in ice pop molds overnight, and serve up delicious treats the next day!

½ cup (125 g) *Kale, Banana, and Hemp Seed Purée*, page 43
1 cup (175 g) quinoa, uncooked, rinsed
1 cup (235 ml) water
1 cup (235 ml) vegetable broth
1 teaspoon butter

1. Combine the quinoa, water, vegetable broth, and butter in a medium saucepan. Bring to a boil. Reduce heat, cover, and simmer on low for 10 minutes, or until the quinoa is fluffy.

2. Mix in *Kale, Banana, and Hemp Seed Purée*. Serve warm.

RECIPE NOTE

....

You can serve this dish with a side of roasted veggies, such as zucchini, carrots, onions, garlic, and potatoes. This is the perfect warm meal after a long day of playing. It is satisfying and leaves your family feeling very full and happy.

Fun Cheddar Crisp Crackers

14+ months

YIELD: ABOUT 5 CUPS (875 G) OF CRACKERS

....

Everyone loves cheesy crackers, and they are usually something we buy boxed at the store for our kid's lunches. However, it's super easy and fun to make your own. Let your kids help with this one. They think it's awesome that they made crackers they can put into their lunch and tell their friends about.

1 stick (½ cup or 112 g) unsalted butter, softened

1 cup (120 g) shredded sharp cheddar cheese

1 cup (245 g) Millet and Cheddar Purée, page 44

1½ cups (185 g) all-purpose flour

1 teaspoon (6 g) sea salt

1. Preheat oven to 325°F (170°C, or gas mark 3).
2. In a food processor, blend all ingredients together to form a ball of dough.
3. Place dough on a floured surface and knead into a ball.
4. Let the dough ball sit in the refrigerator for about 15 minutes.
5. Roll the dough out very thin, approximately ⅛-inch (3 mm)-thick.
6. Using either a pizza cutter or small shaped cookie cutters, cut the dough into cracker squares or shapes. If using a pizza cutter, make the cracker squares about 1½ x 1½-inch (3.8 x 3.8 cm) squares.
7. Bake on a parchment-lined cookie sheet for 10 to12 minutes, until browned.
8. Let sit until fully cooled before serving.

Eggplant Salsa

14+ months

YIELD: ABOUT 2 CUPS (520 G)

....

Every party needs salsa, and this is a fun and unique way to make a healthier version. I also like to give this to my kids in their school lunches with some veggie tortilla chips. Adjust the spice for your children's tastes.

1½ cups (375 g) Roasted Eggplant Purée, page 45

¼ cup (40 g) minced yellow onion

1 garlic clove, minced

¼ cup (4 g) fresh minced cilantro

3 plum tomatoes, finely chopped

2 tablespoons (8 g) fresh minced parsley

1 teaspoon sea salt

1 teaspoon pepper

1 dash of cayenne pepper

1. In a medium sized mixing bowl, combine the *Roasted Eggplant Purée* with all of the other ingredients.
2. Mix well and serve with crackers.

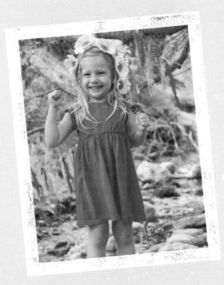

Parmesan Crusted Halibut with Lemon-Caper Sauce

15+ months

YIELD: 4 ADULT SERVINGS OR 6 KID SERVINGS

Halibut is a delicate fish that is great for kids because it's not "fishy" tasting, and its mild flavor is easily complimented by various flavors. The parmesan potato crust is delicious with this fish.

FOR THE HALIBUT:
4 fillets of fresh wild caught halibut
¼ teaspoon each salt and pepper per fillet
1 cup (245 g) *Parmesan Potato Purée* (page 46), divided
2 tablespoons (28 g) unsalted butter

FOR THE SAUCE:
2 lemons, juiced
1 tablespoon (9 g) capers
¼ cup (55 g) butter, melted
salt and pepper, to taste

1. Preheat oven to 350°F (180°C, or gas mark 4).
2. Salt and pepper each piece of fish on both sides, then coat one side of each piece of fish with some of the *Parmesan Potato Purée*, about ¼ cup (60 g) per fillet.
3. Heat up a non-stick skillet. Place butter in the pan. Place each piece of fish, purée side down, into the heated sauté pan and cook for about 5 minutes. Carefully turn over to make sure the crust is intact and cook for an additional 3 minutes.
4. Transfer fish to a baking dish and place in oven for an additional 5 minutes.
5. Meanwhile, in a small saucepan, melt butter. Add in capers, lemon juice, salt, and pepper.
6. Drizzle butter sauce over the top of each piece of fish upon serving.

Apricot and Raspberry Fruit Leather

20+ months

YIELD: ABOUT 30 LEATHERS

Fruit leathers are great for school lunches and after school snacks and are super easy to make. You can adapt this recipe to any one of your fruit purées. I have to admit that I like snacking on these too, and it feels like a treat to my kids. Try turning one of the veggie/fruit purées into these roll ups!

4 cups (1 kg) *Apricot Raspberry Purée*, page 47
2 tablespoons (42 g) raw agave nectar

1. Preheat oven to 120°F (48°C) (or lowest temperature available for your oven).
2. Cover a sheet pan with a piece of heat-resistant plastic wrap or sprayed parchment paper.
3. Combine the *Apricot Raspberry Purée* with the agave nectar.
4. Pour the mixture on the prepared sheet pan in a very thin layer, about ¼-inch (6 mm)-thick.
5. Bake, with oven door left slightly ajar for about 3 hours until fruit purée has dried.
6. Remove from oven and cut with a pizza cutter into long strips, the full length of the pan. Cut those strips in half, and finish up by rolling them. Store in an airtight glass jar.

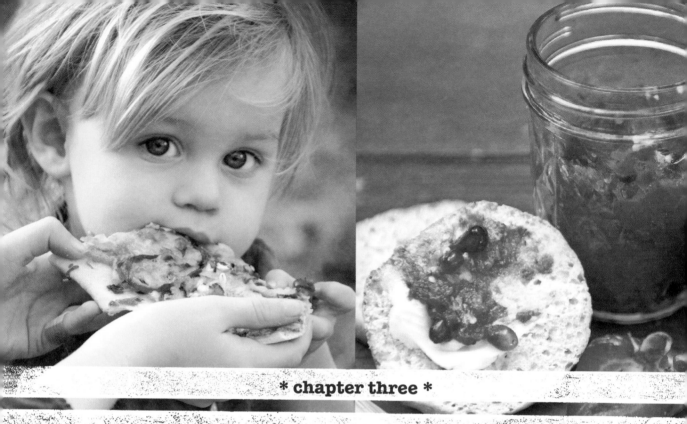

summer purées

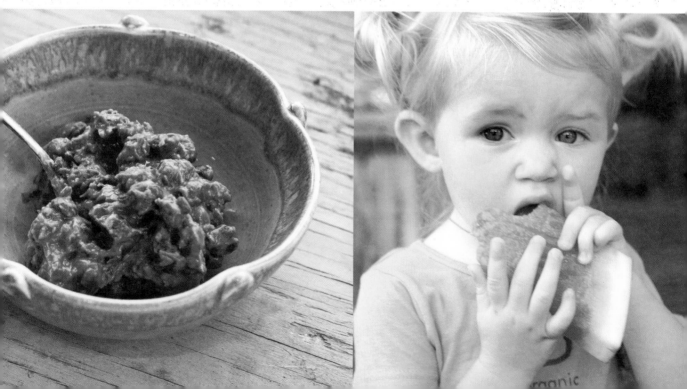

Summer is filled with the bounty of juicy strawberries, peaches, watermelons, berries, and tropical fruits. It is a time to play in the sprinklers, dig in the dirt exploring ladybugs and worms, and watch babies stumble down the wet sand at the beach. We spend a lot of time in our own backyards having BBQs, eating popsicles, and enjoying warm evening dinner parties with friends. Preparing baby food in the summer is just straight up fun! There are so many delicious goodies that nature hands us on a silver platter that it's almost criminal *not* to take advantage of this bounty.

Local and Organic

Eating locally supports our health in many ways. First, eating local means eating seasonal, which means you are eating what your body needs at certain times of the year. Ever wonder why pomegranates are only in season in the fall? In the fall, it starts to get chilly; we start catching little ailments and need extra boosts of vitamins. Along comes superfood, antioxidant, immunity-boosting pomegranates to save the day! When we eat these and other items in season, we give our bodies the benefit of fighting off nature's colds, flus, and other little bugs that pop up *naturally*.

Organic food is not only for health-conscious folks. It's for everyone. When feeding a baby, you are starting her brand new digestive system off with first tastes of nature's goodness, so why not give her the best the Earth has to offer? If you grow a baby food garden, you know for sure that everything in there is as pure as it can be. Even if you do not have a baby food garden and choose a CSA share, a farmer's market, or a grocery store to buy produce, make sure these first picks are as pure and as sweet as the season you are in.

Although we do not know all of the effects spraying chemicals on our food, we do know that higher nitrate content is found in chemically sprayed food, it does not taste as good. Moreover, babies' digestive systems are delicate and are more susceptible to the negative effects of chemicals. Staying away from chemicals is good advice for us all, not just babies. Organic food that has been properly cared for by our farmers is more delicious and juicy, feels better to eat, and is better for the environment.

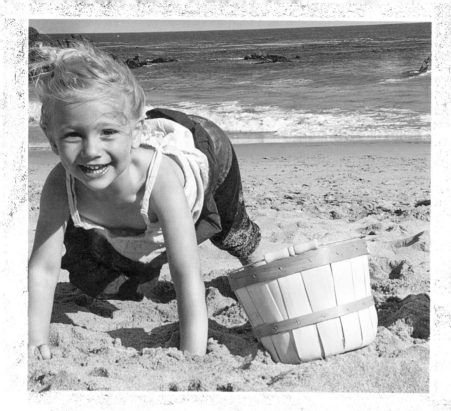
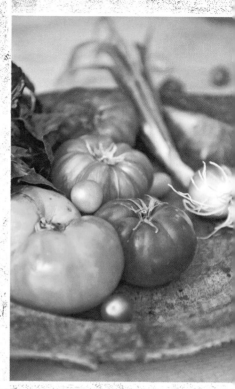

Take Your "Shopping" to the Source!

When teaching our children about food, we should start with the source, our farmers. All food comes from somewhere, and someone has to care for it, grow it, harvest it, and get it to the people. Our farmers do not get the credit they deserve. Getting to know who grows our food can help families find a deeper appreciation for what they put in their bodies. CSAs are popping up all around the country and help support farmers by cutting out the middleman.

How do CSAs work? CSAs enable consumers to buy a share of a local farmer's crop. In return, you pick up fresh fare every week. Participating in a CSA is a great way to eat locally, support sustainable farming and agriculture, and eat seasonally. If the zucchini crop is good, that is what you get. If the corn fails because of too much rain, then you don't get the corn. Many people are used to going to the store to buy all their food and expect to get whatever they want when they want it.

"Shopping" at a CSA may be new to you, but it is a fantastic way to eat the best fresh foods without having to grow it yourself. Farmers are the heroes of the food chain and need to be supported. Organic farmers have an especially tough task, as they fight off critters, bugs, weather, and any other hindrances without the use of toxic chemicals.

Getting your kids excited about going to their CSA every week can help them learn about where their food comes from and who grows it. Seeing my children shake the hand of the farmer who grew the broccoli we used to make the soup we had for dinner brings me such joy, and I know this process will have a lasting effect on them for the rest of their lives.

Farming with Kids

When you teach your children about farming, you are giving them a gift. Specifically, it is a gift of sustainable living and empowerment. A child who knows how to use the land to grow food becomes a resourceful adult who has respect for the bounty of the Earth and can take care of himself. This practice has been lost over the years, and our children not only do not know where their food comes from, but they are totally disconnected from the experience as they go to the store with their parents to buy their food.

Shopping at grocery stores is a reality of course, but if we can include our children in more gardening and farming jobs, it gives them a deeper connection to their own health and nutrition. Start small with a little herb garden if you can, and slowly add things like tomatoes, onions, and other well-used basics.

Picky Eaters

On average, a baby needs to try a new food eight times to develop a liking for the flavor. Babies inherently trust us, so it's important to use that early trust to offer foods that you really want them to eat. Keep in mind that your baby, while he trusts you, is a different person than you and may have likes and dislikes that are different from yours. Many parents make the mistake of not offering foods to their babies that they do not like, thinking their babies will also not like them. However, many times the opposite is true. For example, I do not care for black beans, but I offered them to all my children knowing how good they are for them, and it turns out black beans are two of my children's favorite food.

As your baby grows and enters the toddler years, you may find that he begins a new phase of pickiness. If this is the case, do not despair. There are ways to help your children move through this phase. They will go back to liking a wide range of foods even if it takes awhile. It's important not to give up! Try allowing older children in the home to offer food to your toddlers, or try changing the venue of where they eat, such as outside on the grass on a warm evening. Offering your baby a wide variety of flavors and foods right out of the gate is a good idea, as you naturally form a more diverse culinary palate for him and help him to truly embrace the joy of eating.

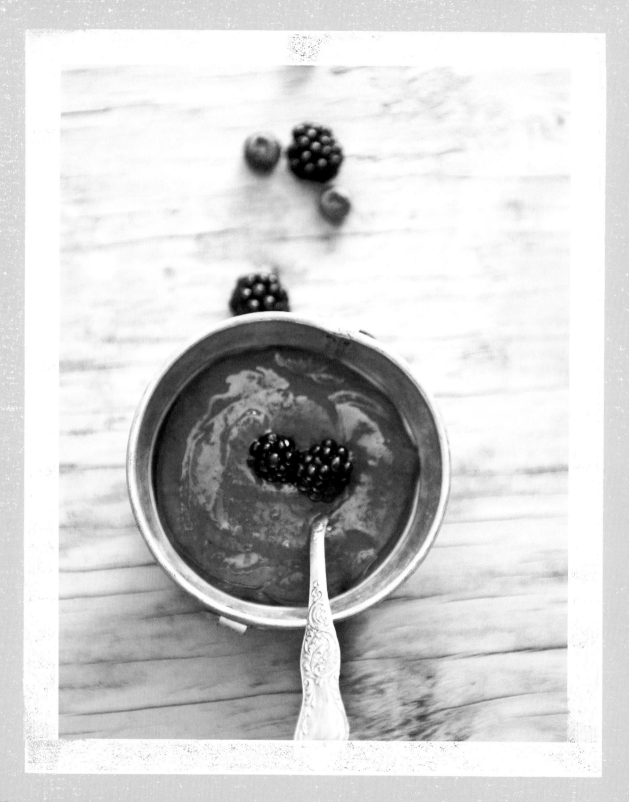

Bountiful Baby Purées

Blackberry-Blueberry Yogurt

8+ months

YIELD: 2 CUPS (460 G), OR 6 TO 8 BABY SERVINGS

2-IN-1 OPTION: **HAM AND BERRY PANINI WITH GOAT CHEESE,** PAGE 90

Yogurt is fabulous for babies, as it is full of live cultures and fats that help with brain development. My babies always love the berry combinations, and my family loves putting a little on sandwiches for a special touch.

½ cup (75 g) whole blueberries
½ cup (75 g) whole blackberries
Purified water for mixing
½ cup (115 g) plain Greek yogurt

1. Wash berries with water and steam for 3 to 5 minutes, until the berries are soft.
2. Press steamed berries through a fine sieve to separate seeds, collecting the juice and pulp in a mixing bowl. Be sure to scrape all of the berry pulp off the bottom of the sieve.
3. Reserve the water from the steamer.
4. Blend the juice and pulp mixture in a blender until puréed. Add 1 teaspoon (5 ml) of reserved water at a time, if necessary, until desired consistency is achieved.
5. Transfer the berry mixture to a mixing bowl, add the yogurt, and whisk until fully combined.

summer purées

Raw Mango, Papaya, and Coconut Purée

7+ months

YIELD: 2 CUPS (490 G), OR 6 TO 8 BABY SERVINGS

2-IN-1 OPTION: **HONEY WONTONS WITH TROPICAL FILLING,** PAGE 91

Babies need a lot of iron, and mangoes are full of not only iron, but antioxidants as well. Combine them with juicy papaya (which is great for digestion) and coconut (which is high in the omega-6 fatty acids that help with brain development), and this becomes a tropical treat worth gobbling up.

1 whole mango
½ papaya
¼ cup (20 g) fresh coconut flakes

1. Peel and cut mango and papaya into chunks.
2. In a blender or food processor, combine mango, papaya, and coconut flakes and blend to desired consistency.
3. Serve cold.

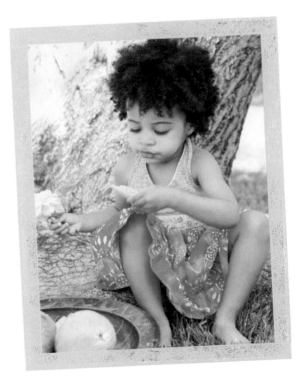

Strawberry, Peach, Pineapple, and Pomegranate Purée

10+ months

YIELD: 4 CUPS (980 G), OR 8 BABY SERVINGS

2-IN-1 OPTION: **SUMMER LOVIN' YOGURT CRUNCH,** PAGE 91

The tropical flavors of this purée mixture are loved by all babies. It's super high in antioxidants and has a sweet and tart flavor profile. Make this recipe toward the very end of the summer, when pomegranates are just beginning to come into season (which extends through fall), and you will be able to grab all the natural sweetness from each fruit.

2 cups (350 g) chopped strawberries
2 cups (300 g) chopped peaches (skin on is fine)
1 small pineapple, skinned and chopped into chunks
1 cup (175 g) fresh pomegranate seeds

1. Combine all ingredients in a blender and purée until well blended. If desired, add in 1 teaspoon of water at time to get the purée to a smoother consistency.

Pure Peach Purée

6+ months

YIELD: 3 CUPS (750 G), OR 8 BABY SERVINGS

2-IN-1 OPTION: **HOMEMADE PEACH MINT ICE CREAM,** PAGE 92

In the summer, peaches are nature's candy. This stone fruit is sweet and delicious and a great first food for your baby. Peaches are high in vitamins C and A, high in fiber, easy to digest, and considered a low allergen fruit.

5 whole peaches

1. Wash and cut peaches, leaving skins on.
2. Steam the peaches for 5 to 7 minutes, until soft. Reserve the cooking water from the steamer.
3. Transfer the peaches to a food processor, and add 2 tablespoons (28 ml) of the reserved water.
4. Purée until smooth.

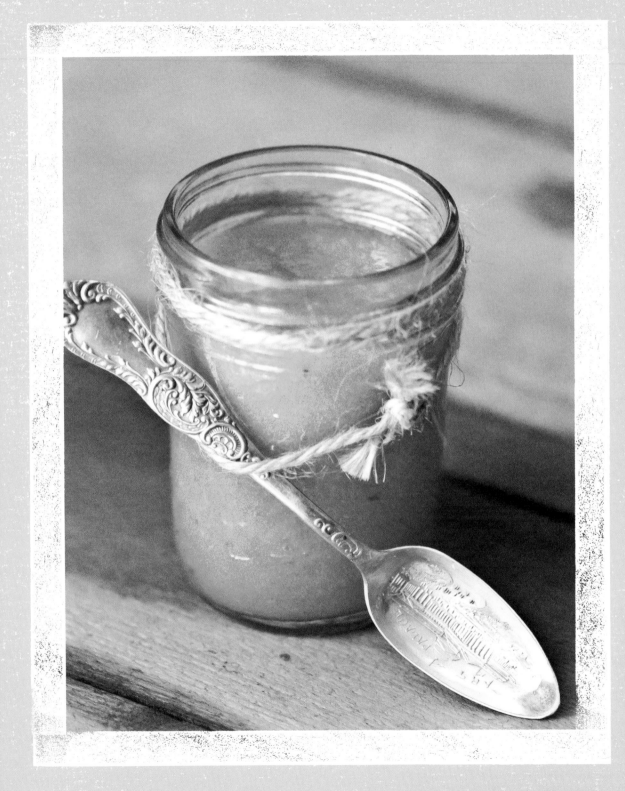

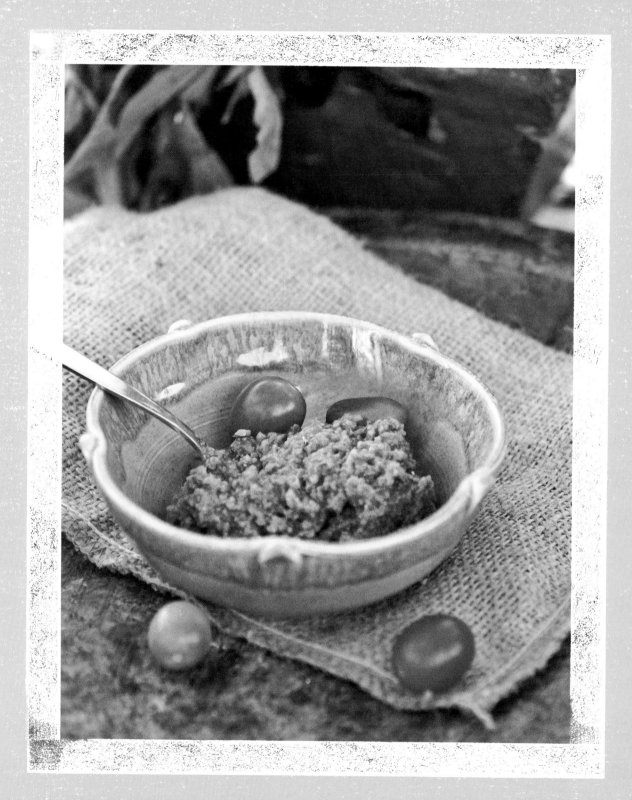

Roasted Tomato, Kale, and Garlic Textured Purée

9+ months

YIELD: 3 CUPS (750 G), OR 8 BABY SERVINGS

2-IN-1 OPTION: **PERFECT ROASTED TOMATO SOUP,** PAGE 93

Tomatoes are high in vitamin C, while kale is full of vitamins K, A, and C. Together, they make a flavor packed purée that babies love. When they get a little older and want texture, try throwing this purée over mini-pasta or mixed in with millet or quinoa—the whole family will enjoy.

2 large tomatoes, cut in half
2 large garlic cloves
1 tablespoon (15 ml) olive oil
1 cup (75 g) fresh kale leaves, stems removed

1. Preheat oven to 300°F (150° C).
2. On a parchment-lined baking tray, place tomatoes and peeled garlic and lightly drizzle with olive oil. Roast in the oven for 15 minutes.
3. Steam the kale until soft, about 5 to 7 minutes.
4. Combine the roasted tomatoes, garlic, and kale in the blender or food processor and purée until smooth. Serve warm.

summer purées

Strawberry and Plum Purée

9+ months

YIELD: 2 CUPS (500 G), OR 5 BABY SERVINGS

2-IN-1 OPTION: **BEST BUTTERMILK BISCUITS AND SUMMER JAM**, PAGE 94

Strawberries and plums are a dream combination for a baby and for a cook. This sweet dynamo lends itself to lots of potential dishes, but babies absolutely love this nature's candy. Strawberries are considered a citrus that is also a higher allergen, so waiting until your baby is a little older is better as their digestive tracts get more mature and able to handle more foods. Strawberries and plums are both high in vitamin C, and plums are also high in potassium.

3 plums, peeled and cubed
2 cups (350 g) chopped strawberries

1. Steam plums and strawberries together for 5 to 7 minutes, until they are soft. Reserve the water from the steamer.
2. Blend the plum-strawberry mixture in a blender until puréed. Add 1 teaspoon of reserved water at a time, if necessary, until desired consistency is achieved.

summer purées

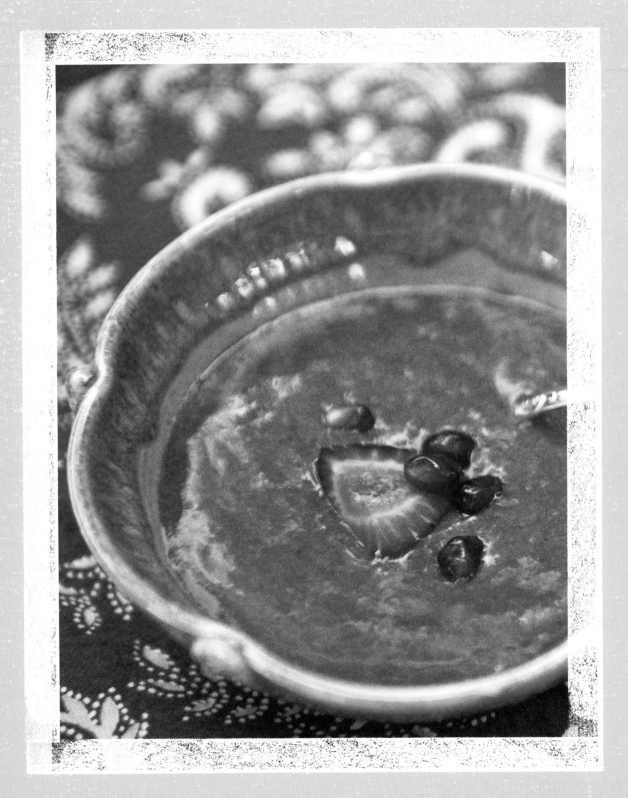

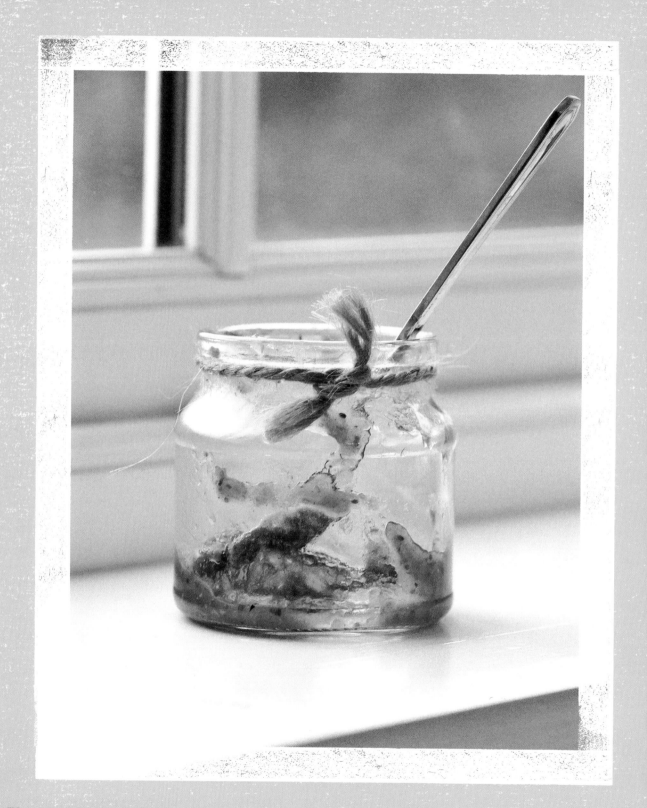

Bountiful Baby Purées

Strawberry, Fig, and Banana Purée

9+ months

YIELD: 2 CUPS (500 G), OR 4 BABY SERVINGS

2-IN-1 OPTION: **STRAWBERRY TURNOVERS WITH LEMON-INFUSED WHIPPED CREAM AND FIG DRIZZLE, PAGE 95**

....

Figs are delicious! They seem somewhat exotic to me, but they are just a simple fruit that many folks don't know what to do with. They have a natural sticky sweetness that is somewhat nutty in flavor and are high in potassium and fiber. They grow on trees and are part of the Mulberry family. They are also a great after school snack drizzled with warmed honey and served with cheese and crackers.

2 cups (350 g) chopped strawberries
4 fresh figs, halved
2 bananas, peeled and sliced

1. Steam strawberries and figs together for 3 minutes, until they are soft.
2. Reserve the water from the steamer.
3. Blend the strawberry–fig mixture with the bananas in a blender until puréed.
4. Add 1 teaspoon (5 ml) of reserved water at a time, if necessary, until desired consistency is achieved.

RECIPE NOTE

....

You can make this recipe with dried figs, but they are smaller, so use six instead of four.

Spinach, Basil, and Wheat Germ Pesto Purée

12+ months

YIELD: 1½ CUPS (500 G), OR 3 BABY SERVINGS

2-IN-1 OPTION: **SUMMER VEGGIE FLATBREAD PESTO PIZZA,** PAGE 96

....

Adding herbs to your baby food creations is a wonderful way to introduce unique flavors and aromatics. This is a great recipe for your baby as he starts to be able to handle more texture. You can pour this pesto over tiny pastas or orzo for your growing adventurous eater.

3 cups (100 g) of spinach, chopped
2 cups (80 g) fresh basil, chopped
1 large garlic clove, minced
¼ cup (50 g) fresh grated Parmesan cheese
¼ cup (33 g) pine nuts or walnuts
1 tablespoon (7 g) wheat germ
¼ cup (60 ml) olive oil

1. Combine the spinach, basil, garlic, cheese, nuts, and wheat germ in a food processor or blender and purée.

2. Slowly stream in the olive oil while puréeing.

3. Feed to baby as a purée or serve over tiny pasta or orzo if your baby is eating textured meals.

summer purées

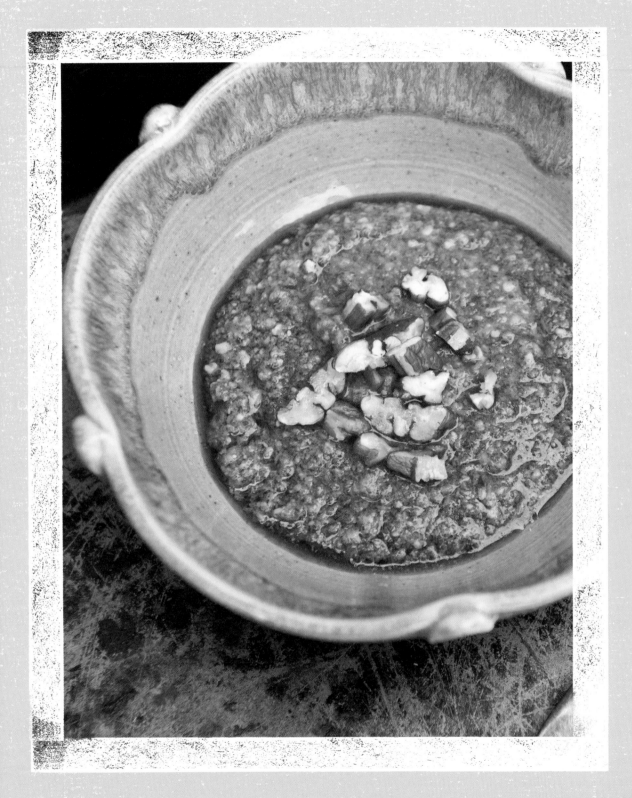

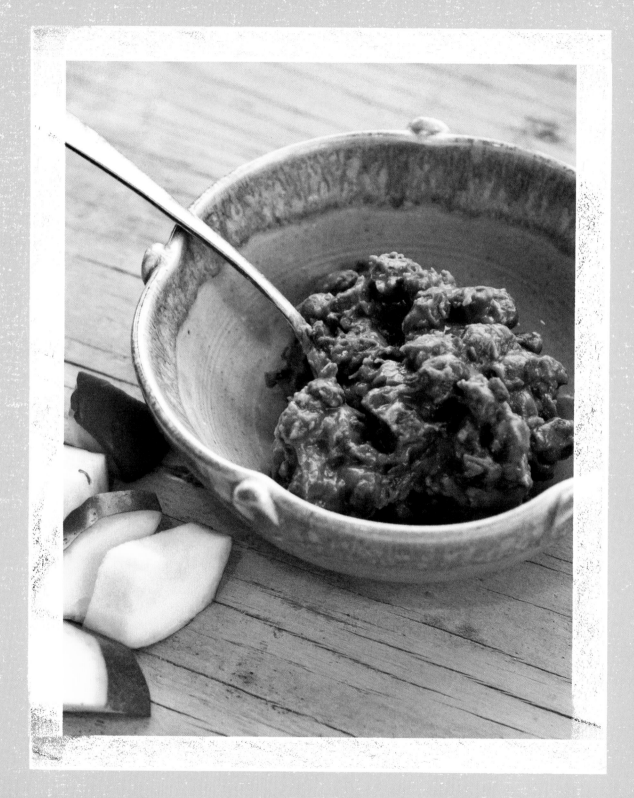

Slow Cooker Black Beans, Zucchini, and Feta Cheese Blend

11+ months

YIELD: 10 CUPS (2.5 TO 3 KG), OR 20 BABY SERVINGS

2-IN-1 OPTION: **WHOLE WHEAT BLACK BEAN QUESADILLAS,** PAGE 97

Black beans are filled with protein and packed with flavor. My baby River goes crazy for black beans. When you offer them with a little feta cheese, it deepens the flavor profile and helps your newly chewing baby practice! Making this dish in the slow cooker makes it little work for you; all it takes is a little preplanning.

1 pound (450 g) fresh black beans, washed and soaked
32 ounces (1 kg) chicken stock
2 bay leaves
1 onion, chopped
2 cloves of garlic, chopped
2 zucchinis, chopped
½ cup (75 g) feta cheese

1. Soak beans in water overnight
2. The next day, drain your beans and place them to your slow cooker. Cover them with chicken stock.
3. Add onion, garlic, zucchini, and feta cheese.
4. Cook overnight (roughly 8 hours) on high. Meal will be ready to enjoy in the morning.

summer purées

Thai Coconut Rice Textured Meal

11+ months

YIELD: 2 CUPS (350 G), OR 4 BABY SERVINGS

2-IN-1 OPTION: **COCONUT SHRIMP SOUP,** PAGE 98

This classic Thai dish is tasty and fun. It gives your growing child a chance to try new foods. If your baby is not chewing great by now, pulse this dish in the blender after it's completed to make it a little less textured and easier to chew.

2 cups (475 ml) coconut milk
¼ teaspoon (2.2 g) turmeric
1 cup (200 g) basmati rice, uncooked
1 yellow onion, minced small
1 garlic clove, minced
¼ teaspoon Bragg Liquid Aminos

1. In a medium saucepan, warm the coconut milk and turmeric together. Add the rice, onion, garlic, and liquid aminos. Stir and cover.

2. Bring to a boil, then reduce heat, keeping the lid on and let simmer for about 10 minutes, or until the rice is tender. Be careful not to overcook the rice.

3. Serve warm.

Veggie Ratatouille

11+ months

YIELD: 4 CUPS (1 KG), OR 8 BABY SERVINGS

2-IN-1 OPTION: **MAMA AND PAPA RATATOUILLE,** PAGE 99

This is a classic dish that gives your baby all kinds of garden goodness in one meal. It's fun to have a tasty dish that uses every leftover vegetable. My son Bodhi used to love this dish as a baby, and I always felt so good being able to grab most of the ingredients straight from my garden. If you plan on making a portion of this into the *Mama and Papa Ratatouille,* reserve 3 cups (730 g) before blending.

2 tablespoons (30 ml) coconut oil

1 yellow onion, chopped

1 garlic clove, minced

1 teaspoon fresh oregano

2 cups (375 g) cubed Roma tomatoes

1 zucchini, peeled and cubed

1 yellow bell pepper, cubed

1 small purple eggplant, peeled and cubed

½ teaspoon fresh rosemary

½ cup (20 g) fresh basil

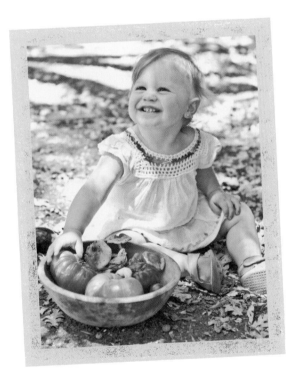

1. In a large pot, heat the coconut oil. Add the onion, garlic, and oregano and sauté until lightly browned.

2. Add tomatoes, zucchini, bell pepper, eggplant, rosemary, and basil and stew on medium heat until vegetables are softened and flavors are well blended.

3. Put the entire vegetable medley in the blender and hit pulse until you reached the desired consistency.

Spinach, Kale, Broccoli, Goji, and Banana Purée

7+ months

YIELD: 2 CUPS (500 G), OR 4 BABY SERVINGS

2-IN-1 OPTION: **BACKYARD BBQ TURKEY BURGERS,** PAGE 99

This purée is a powerhouse of nutrition and is filled with super antioxidants and proteins. The stand-out ingredient is the goji berries. If you are not familiar with this dried fruit treat, goji berries are high in immunity-building properties and vitamin C. They are widely available now and can be purchased at your local health food store.

1 cup (70 g) chopped broccoli
1 cup (30 g) spinach leaves, packed, stems removed
1 cup (30 g) kale leaves, chopped and packed, stems removed
½ cup (75 g) goji berries
2 bananas, peeled and sliced

1. Steam broccoli, spinach, kale, and goji berries together for 3 to 5 minutes, until they are soft. Reserve the water from the steamer.

2. Blend the mixture in a blender with the banana slices until puréed. Add 1 teaspoon of reserved water at a time, if necessary, until desired consistency is achieved.

summer purées

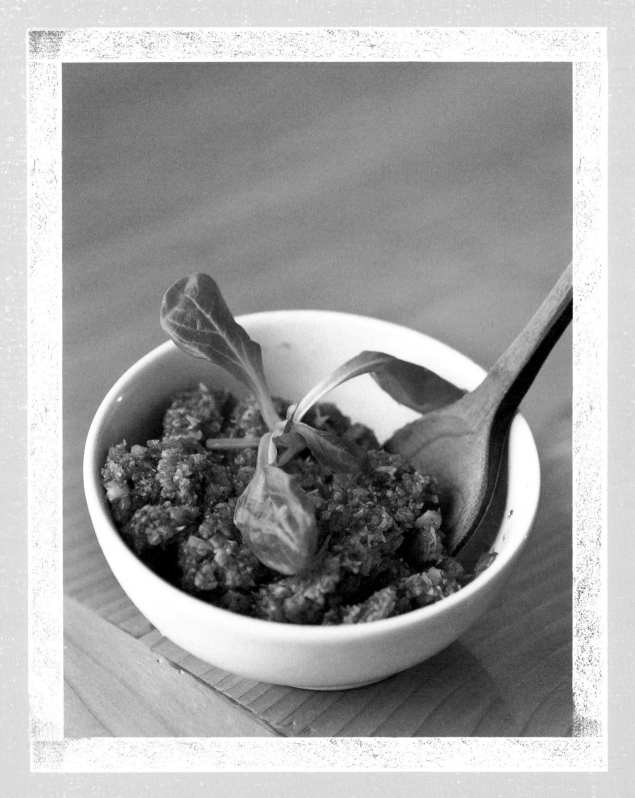

Slow Cooker Steel-Cut Oats and Berries

9+ months

YIELD: 4 CUPS, OR 6 TO 8 BABY SERVINGS

2-IN-1 OPTION: **NOURISHING BERRY OATMEAL CAKE,** PAGE 100

Oats are a wonderfully satisfying meal, and babies love them. Using the whole grain preserves the nutritional value, and making oats in a slow cooker allows you the benefit of dumping and going. For busy parents, that is a great alternative, especially if your family is anything like ours and there is a need to feed a bunch of little ones first thing in the morning before school.

1 cup (80 g) steel-cut oats, uncooked
4½ cups (1 L) water
1 cup (125 g) raspberries
½ teaspoon wheat germ

1. Combine all ingredients into a lightly greased, large slow cooker.
2. Cook on low overnight, 6 to 8 hours.

Pizza Party Purée

11+ months

YIELD: 2½ CUPS (600 G), OR 4 TO 5 BABY SERVINGS

2-IN-1 OPTION: **FRIENDS AND FAMILY PIZZA,** PAGE 100

Who doesn't like a pizza party? They are a great way to come together and share food. This purée makes a great dipping sauce too. All of my kids used to love to grab a hold of a bread stick and dip into the sauce. Homemade teething biscuits make great dippers, too!

1 tablespoon (15 ml) coconut oil
1 medium yellow onion, chopped
1 garlic clove, minced
1 teaspoon fresh oregano
3 carrots, peeled and chopped
2 cups (360 g) cubed Roma tomatoes
½ cup (20 g) fresh basil

1. In a large pot, heat the coconut oil. Add the onion, garlic, oregano, and carrots and sauté until the onions are golden brown and the carrots are soft.

2. Add tomatoes and basil and stew on medium heat until vegetables are softened and flavors are well blended.

3. Put the entire mixture in the blender and hit pulse until you reach the desired consistency.

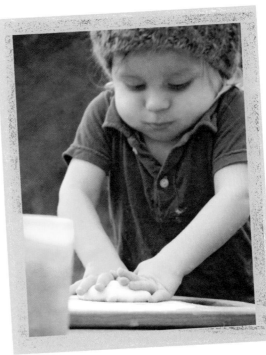

summer purées

Crab, Lemon, and Bell Pepper Textured Meal

12+ months

YIELD: 2 CUPS (500 G), OR 4 BABY SERVINGS

2-IN-1 OPTION: **ZESTY CRAB CAKES**, PAGE 101

This little gem of a recipe is just getting your baby's feet wet, so to speak, in the world of crab and summer cookouts. Wait until your baby is ready to dig in with a healthy appetite and some chewing ability before offering this one. Please don't throw any of it out though; this mixture can be magically transformed into delicious crab cakes for everyone!

½ **small red bell pepper, chopped in long slices**
½ **pound (8 ounces or 225 g) lump crab, picked over**
2 **tablespoons (30 ml) lemon juice**

1. Preheat oven to 350°F (180°C, or gas mark 4).
2. Place the red bell pepper pieces in a glass shallow baking dish and roast for 15 to 20 minutes.
3. Combine the roasted pepper with the crab and lemon and pulse in the blender until desired texture consistency is achieved.

Rainbow Eating

When feeding your baby, it's important to keep color in mind. Eating a rainbow of colorful foods is the easiest way to quickly make sure that your baby is getting all the nutritional variety he needs. Your baby's plate should always have beautiful colors represented, such as greens, yellows, oranges, reds, and purples. Embracing the rainbow is a great way to naturally support seasonal and local eating.

Pure Nectarine Purée

6+ months

YIELD: 3 CUPS (750 G), OR 8 BABY SERVINGS

2-IN-1 OPTION: **NECTARINE TEETHING BISCUITS,** PAGE 101

Similar to the peach, this stone fruit is sweet and delicious when in season, and it is a wonderfully easy first food for babies to digest. I love this fruit for jams, pies, and summer salads, but I could eat bushes of plain, fresh nectarines. Babies naturally love this sweet purée, which is a good thing because it's rich in vitamins A and C, among other valuable nutrients.

5 whole nectarines

1. Wash and cut nectarines, leaving skins on.
2. Steam the nectarines for 5 to 7 minutes, or until soft. Reserve the cooking water from the steamer.
3. Transfer the nectarines to a food processor, and add in 2 tablespoons (28 ml) of the reserved water.
4. Purée until desired consistency is achieved.

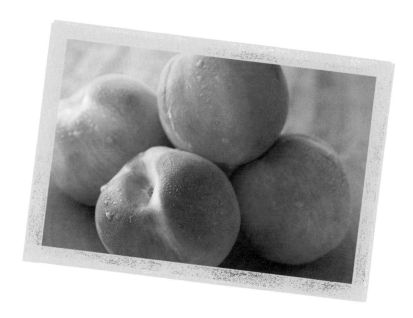

Ham and Berry Panini with Goat Cheese

15+ months

YIELD: 2 ADULT SERVINGS OR 4 KID SERVINGS

....

This sweet and savory combination is a delicious twist on a classic ham 'n cheese sandwich. It's also fun for kids to help assemble—especially once they learn that there are some flowers you can eat. Note that you will need a panini press to make this dish.

4 slices sourdough bread (use your favorite)
A few slices of your favorite ham
2 tablespoons (20 g) goat cheese
2 tablespoons (30 g) *Blackberry-Blueberry Yogurt*, page 67
Salad greens with edible flowers

1. Preheat your panini press.
2. Assemble your sandwiches by spreading two of the slices with the goat cheese, and two with the *Blackberry-Blueberry Yogurt*.
3. Layer ham on goat cheese side of bread, and top with remaining bread slices (yogurt side facing down). Place on panini press and let cheese melt. Flip sandwich once or twice.
4. After the sandwich has been grilled, open up and add your greens and edible flowers (this keeps the sandwich tasting fresh). Serve immediately.

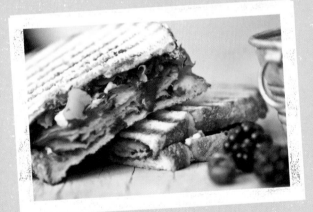

EDIBLE FLOWERS!
....

Did you know there are certain types of flowers you can eat? Squash blossoms, nasturtiums, lavender, chamomile, chive blossoms, basil, dandelions, fennel, violets, and pumpkin blossom are edible, to name a few. Remember that not all flowers are edible, so check before you eat them and make sure they have not been sprayed with pesticides. Adding these pretty flowers to sandwiches and salads is fun, vibrant, and delicious.

Honey Wontons with Tropical Filling

12+ months

YIELD: MAKES 16 WONTONS, OR SERVINGS

....

Wontons are fun to eat and are great finger foods for toddlers. I call this recipe dessert in my house because my kids love to have a little extra honey as a dipping sauce. It's a treat that you can feel good about serving up to your little ones.

1 (16 ounces) package of wonton wrappers, makes 16 wontons

3 tablespoons (60 g) honey

1 cup (250 g) *Raw Mango, Papaya, and Coconut Purée*, page 68

3 tablespoons (100 g) chopped pistachios

1 tablespoon (8 g) sesame seeds

1. Preheat oven to 350°F (180° C).
2. Place wonton wrappers on a flat surface, and brush the whole inside of each one with honey.
3. Put one teaspoon (5 ml) of the *Raw Mango, Papaya, and Coconut Purée* and a few chopped pistachios onto the center of each wrapper.
4. Moisten edges of wrappers with wet fingers, then fold over to form a triangle.
5. Press edges together to seal.
6. Sprinkle the top of each wonton with sesame seeds.
7. Bake on a baking sheet lined with parchment paper for about 15 minutes, until they are golden brown.

Summer Lovin' Yogurt Crunch

13+ months

YIELD: 2 TO 3 CUPS (500 TO 750 G), OR 4 TO 6 SERVINGS

....

This recipe makes for a wonderful breakfast or great on-the-go snack. I find that when you make your own yogurt combinations, they are always far superior to the ones you buy at the store. First, they are not overly sweet and second, you can be creative with your mix-ins. Have fun creating all kinds of combos!

1 cup plain Greek yogurt

1½ cups (375 g) *Strawberry, Peach, Pineapple, and Pomegranate Purée*, page 69

1 teaspoon ground flaxseed

½ cup (60 g) your favorite granola mixture

1. Gently combine all ingredients in a bowl and serve immediately.

RECIPE NOTES

....

> If serving this to your little one, be sure to chop the granola up so there are no large chunks. You can also add a small amount of purified water if the mixture seems too thick.
> Instead of combining everything together at once, layer the ingredients, parfait-style, into small bowls or glasses and have kids mix their own.

Homemade Peach Mint Ice Cream

12+ months

1½ QUARTS (575 G), OR 8 SERVINGS

Who doesn't love creamy homemade ice cream? This is a wonderful summer treat for the whole family. By making it yourself, you are in charge of the ingredients. You might consider using this for baby's first taste of ice cream on his birthday! Note that you will need an ice cream maker to prepare this dish.

2 eggs
1 cup (340 g) raw agave nectar
½ cup (100 g) pure cane sugar
1 teaspoon (5 ml) vanilla extract
2 tablespoons (28 ml) freshly squeezed lemon juice
2 drops of pure mint extract
3 cups (750 g) *Pure Peach Purée*, page 70
2 cups (475 ml) heavy whipping cream
1 cup (235) whole milk

1. Combine eggs, agave, sugar, vanilla, lemon, and mint extract in a medium sized mixing bowl and beat well.
2. Add *Pure Peach Purée*.
3. Add cream and milk and beat until well blended. Chill immediately.
4. Follow the instructions on your ice cream maker for the final steps.

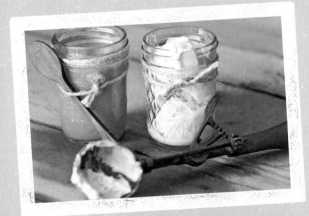

EGG EDUCATION

Make sure you are buying organic eggs that are from free-range chickens. My friend Bobby has a farm near my house called Frog Hollow, and she has more than 300 chickens that are left to roam free during the day and are guarded by herding dogs at night. Her eggs are incredible, and I love supporting a friend and a sustainable practice. The animals are not mistreated, and my family gets fresh, huge eggs. Do not worry about adding raw eggs to this recipe, as it's fine to do, as long as you are careful about your egg choice.

Perfect Roasted Tomato Soup

9+ months

YIELD: 10 CUPS (2.5 L), OR 10 TO 12 SERVINGS

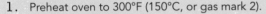

I love tomato soup, and on a chilly autumn day nothing tastes better. I have worked and worked on this soup, and believe I have it perfected now. Of course your baby can also partake and enjoy!

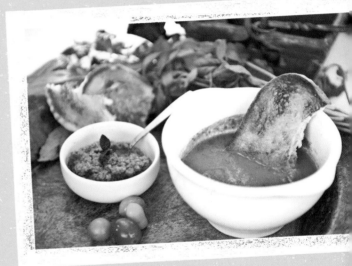

8 large beefsteak tomatoes, washed and sliced in half

6 garlic cloves, peeled

2 tablespoons (28 ml) white wine vinegar

2 pinches sea salt

4 pinches pepper

2 tablespoons (5 g) dried thyme, divided

1 large yellow onion, chopped

1 tablespoon (14 g) unsalted butter

4 cups (1 L) vegetable stock

2 vegetable bouillon cubes

1 cup (250 g) *Roasted Tomato, Kale, and Garlic Textured Purée*, page 73

1 pinch red pepper flakes

Wedges of 2 limes

1. Preheat oven to 300°F (150°C, or gas mark 2).
2. On a parchment-lined baking tray, place halved tomatoes and garlic, and lightly drizzle with vinegar, salt, pepper, and thyme. Roast in the oven for 45 minutes.
3. After the tomatoes have been cooking for 30 minutes, in a large soup pot, melt the butter and sauté the chopped onion until browned. Season with salt, pepper, and thyme.
4. Add the roasted tomatoes and garlic to the pot.
5. Add vegetable stock, bouillons cubes, *Roasted Tomato, Kale, and Garlic Textured Purée*, and red pepper flakes and let simmer for about 5 minutes. Mix well so the flavors meld.
6. Using a hand mixer or blender, purée until soup is a smooth consistency.
7. Squeeze lime wedge on top upon serving.

Best Buttermilk Biscuits and Summer Jam

16+ months

YIELD: 6 TO 8 BISCUITS, OR SERVINGS

Using your purées to make jam is a great way to use up leftovers and give your jam a boost of nutrition. This entire recipe is fun to make with kids, and you might use extras of your sweet summer jam for friendly gifts for your neighbors. Agar is a thickening agent made from seaweed and is a good vegetarian substitute for gelatin. Look for it in health food stores, or online.

FOR JAM:

1 cup (350 g) raw agave nectar

½ cup (100 g) pure cane sugar

1 large lemon, zested and juiced

1 cup fresh chopped strawberries

2 cups (500 g) *Strawberry and Plum Purée*, page 74

1 teaspoon (5 ml) agar

FOR BISCUITS:

2 cups (250 g) all-purpose, self-rising flour

1½ teaspoons (7g) baking powder

½ teaspoon (7 g) baking soda

½ (3 g) teaspoon sea salt

¼ (55 g) cup cold butter, cut into small cubes

¾ cups (175 ml) buttermilk, fresh if possible

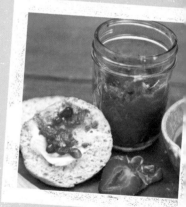

TO MAKE THE JAM:

1. In medium saucepan, combine the agave, sugar, and lemon zest and juice and heat until well combined.

2. Add fresh strawberries and the *Strawberry and Plum Purée*, and let simmer for about 3 minutes. Add in the agar.

3. Let the jam thicken for another 2 minutes and then store in glass jars with airtight lids.

TO MAKE THE BISCUITS:

1. Preheat oven to 500°F (250°C, or gas mark 9). You want a fully hot oven for baking really flaky good biscuits!

2. In a medium-size bowl, blend together flour, baking powder, baking soda, and salt.

3. With a dough hook mixer, cut the butter into the dough until the mixture gets crumby. Stir in the buttermilk and shape the dough into a ball.

4. On a floured work surface, knead the dough until it is smoothly blended. Roll out the dough to about ¾-inch (2 cm)-thick and use a biscuit cutter or glass to cut out biscuits.

5. Brush the tops of the biscuits with melted butter and place them in the center of a baking sheet, sides touching. Bake 8 to 10 minutes or until golden brown.

Strawberry Turnovers with Lemon-Infused Whipped Cream and Fig Drizzle

18+ months

YIELD: 8 TO 10 SERVINGS

....

I love light and flaky pastries. Fill them with all of this goodness and you cannot go wrong. This is another dessert that may seem super fancy, but is actually easy, delicious, and fairly quick to assemble.

6 fresh figs
¼ cup (85 g) raw agave nectar
2 cups (475 ml) heavy whipping cream
1 whole lemon, juiced
3 tablespoons (60 g) honey
1 sheet of puff pastry, chilled, not frozen
1 cup (245 g) *Strawberry, Fig, and Banana Purée*, page 77

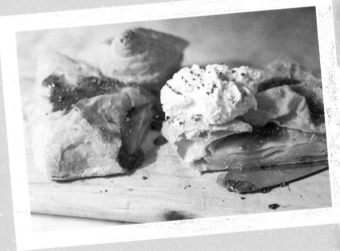

1. Preheat oven to 350°F (180°C, or gas mark 4). Line a cookie sheet with parchment paper.

2. To make the fig drizzle: In a small saucepan, combine the figs and agave nectar and turn the heat to medium while you stir and break down the figs. After 6 to 8 minutes of slow cooking them, mash them together and purée this mixture in your blender. Store in a glass jar on the side.

3. To make the whipped cream: Using a large table top mixer or hand mixer, pour the heavy cream in a bowl, adding the lemon juice and honey. Mix until whipped into a fluffy cream, 4 to 5 minutes. Transfer to a bowl and refrigerate until the puff pastry comes out of the oven.

4. On a floured surface, roll out puff pastry, into a rustic, imperfect circle, about ¼-inch (6-mm) thick. Create an edge on all sides by rolling up some pastry. Poke a fork in the center of the dough a couple of times. Move the dough to the parchment-lined cookie sheet.

5. Spread the *Strawberry, Fig, and Banana Purée* over the top of the puff pastry. Fold over and close the seams in a triangle shape.

6. Bake on the prepared cookie sheet for 15 to 18 minutes until pastry has puffed up and is light and golden brown in color.

7. Serve with chilled whipped cream and warm fig drizzle.

Summer Veggie Flatbread Pesto Pizza

18+ months

YIELD: 4 ADULT SERVINGS, OR 6 KID SERVINGS

This pizza is addictive! This is a fun and easy twist on pizza night and a great way to use any leftover pesto. Basil is filled with anti-bacterial properties, and its classic flavor adds an amazing twist to this dish. Sweet piquanté peppers are also known by the brand name "Peppadew" and can be found jarred—look for them near the pickles.

3 pieces of garlic flatbread
2 cups (500 g) *Spinach, Basil, and Wheat Germ Pesto Purée*, page 78
2 summer heirloom tomatoes, sliced thin, divided
1 cup (150 g) sweet piquanté peppers, chopped, divided
1 small green pepper, sliced thinly, divided
1 small red onion, sliced thin, divided
1 teaspoon (1 g) dried oregano
2 cups (230 g) fresh shredded mozzarella cheese, divided

1. Preheat oven to 425°F (220°C, or gas mark 7).

2. Place flatbreads on a pizza stone or a cookie sheet and bake without any of the toppings for 5 minutes.

3. Remove flatbread from oven and spread S*pinach, Basil, and Wheat Germ Pesto Purée* over the top.

4. Divide tomatoes, both kinds of peppers, red onion, oregano, and cheese over all 3 flatbreads. Drizzle pizzas with a touch of olive oil.

5. Bake flatbreads for 10 to 12 more minutes, until cheese is melted and slightly browned.

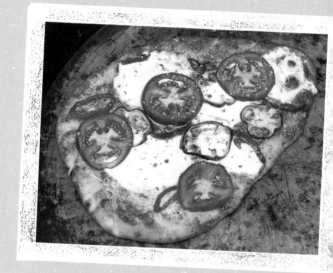

Whole Wheat Black Bean Quesadillas

18+ months

YIELD: 4 ADULT SERVINGS OR 6 KID SERVINGS

This is a super easy and fun dish that uses a lot of healthy beans and can be made in less than 10 minutes. Feel free to swap out the feta with any other cheese you like, along with any additional veggies you have hanging around.

6 whole wheat tortillas

2 cups (500 g) *Slow Cooker Black Beans, Zucchini, and Feta Cheese Blend*, page 81

1 cup (150 g) feta cheese

1. Assemble the quesadilla by laying one plain tortilla out and spreading the *Slow Cooker Black Beans, Zucchini, and Feta Cheese Blend* on top. Add a little bit of feta cheese and place another tortilla on top.

2. Repeat with remaining tortillas.

3. Heat a little olive oil in a medium sized sauté pan on medium heat.

4. Carefully place assembled black bean quesadilla in the pan.

5. Flip twice as the cheese melts and a light crunchy texture develops, about 4 minutes.

6. Cut into triangles and serve warm.

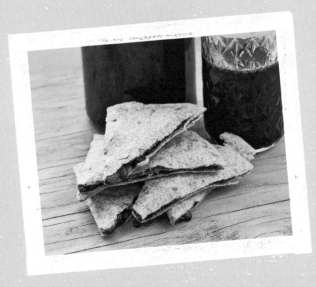

Coconut Shrimp Soup

14+ months

YIELD: 4 CUPS, OR 4 SERVINGS

....

This is a delicious Thai soup that everyone will love—you have to try it! As an alternative to soup, you can serve the shrimp on its own with the Thai Coconut Rice Textured Meal on the side if you like.

1½ pounds (700 g) raw uncooked large shrimp,
   shelled, deveined, and washed in cold water
2 cans (14 ounces, or 425 ml each) coconut milk, divided
¼ teaspoon sea salt
¼ teaspoon pepper
½ cup (8 g) fresh cilantro, minced, divided
2 teaspoons (4 g) freshly ground or minced ginger
2 teaspoons (10 ml) Sriracha (Thai hot chili sauce)
2 tablespoons (28 ml) fish sauce
2 garlic cloves, minced very small
1 cup (245 g) *Thai Coconut Rice Textured Meal*, page 82
1 lemon, juiced
1 tablespoon (14 g) unsalted butter
½ cup (20 g) fresh basil leaves, cut into strips

1. In a large pan, pour ½ cup (120 ml) coconut milk and lay the shrimp in the milk to soak. Season both sides of the shrimp with salt and pepper and add in half of the chopped cilantro.

2. Let the shrimp soak in the mixture while you prepare the soup. After the soup is ready, quickly grill the shrimp.

3. In a big saucepan, pour and mix together the remaining coconut milk and ginger and bring to a boil. Season with salt and pepper.

4. Add the Sriracha, fish sauce, and garlic cloves and stir well.

5. Add the *Thai Coconut Rice Textured Meal*.

6. Let simmer on low while you grill the shrimp.

7. Place the marinated shrimp on a hot grill-top pan or electric grill (discard the coconut milk marinade). Make sure some of the cilantro leaves are on top of each piece. While they are grilling, add a little butter and lemon juice to each piece. Turn after 2 or 3 minutes. Shrimp cooks fast, about 3 minutes on each side, depending on their size.

8. Remove soup from heat and place grilled shrimp on the top.

9. Soup into bowls and top with fresh basil and remaining cilantro.

Mama and Papa Ratatouille

14+ months

YIELD: 3 CUPS (750 G), OR 4 TO 6 SERVINGS

....

If you can serve this meal with a nice side of brown rice, it will be a classic in your home and one you can pull out in a moment's notice. Feel free to substitute vegetables if you are making this dish without having time to properly shop for it.

3 cups (750 g) *Veggie Ratatouille* (page 83), before pulsing it in your blender, if possible

2 tablespoons (28 ml) Bragg liquid aminos

1 tablespoon (15 ml) roasted sesame oil

¼ teaspoon sea salt

¼ teaspoon pepper

1 tablespoon (15 ml) low sodium soy sauce

1. In a wok or large sauté pan, combine the *Veggie Ratatouille* with all of the other ingredients.

2. Sauté over medium heat until all flavors are melded well together.

3. Serve warm with a side of brown rice.

Backyard BBQ Turkey Burgers

15+ months

YIELD: 8 TO 10 BURGERS, OR SERVINGS

....

Try turkey burgers to keep it light and lean during your summer BBQs. Turkey burgers are delicious, and when you add in the power-house purée, they get elevated to super healthy status. Top with fresh greens, Havarti cheese, summer heirloom tomatoes, sliced red onions, and your favorite dressing and you have a fantastic summer meal.

3 pounds (1.5 kg) ground turkey

¼ cup (30 g) panko bread crumbs

1 cup (245 g) *Spinach, Kale, Broccoli, Goji, and Banana Purée*, page 84

½ cup (85 g) organic whole black beans (canned are fine)

2 eggs, lightly beaten

1 clove garlic, peeled and minced

1 teaspoon sea salt

1 teaspoon ground black pepper

Your favorite burger buns

1. In a large bowl, mix ground turkey, bread crumbs, *Spinach, Kale, Broccoli, Goji, and Banana Purée*, black beans, eggs, garlic, salt, and pepper. Form into 10 to 12 patties.

2. Cook the patties in a medium skillet over medium heat, turning once or twice until browned, about 4 minutes on each side.

3. Allow each person to assemble her own burgers based on her likes.

Nourishing Berry Oatmeal Cake

15+ months

YIELD: 6 SERVINGS

Everyone enjoys dessert from time to time, and this version is easy, quick, and tasty. Try this as an alternative for baby's first birthday cake!

½ cup (112 g) unsalted butter, softened
¾ cup (170 g) packed brown sugar
½ cup (170 g) raw agave nectar
2 eggs
1 cup (245 g) *Slow Cooker Steel-Cut Oats and Berries*, page 86
1 teaspoon vanilla extract
1 teaspoon baking soda
½ teaspoon sea salt
1 teaspoon ground cinnamon
1 teaspoon ground flaxseed
1½ cups (187 g) all-purpose flour
½ cup (75 g) raisins
Fresh berries, for serving

1. Preheat oven to 350°F (180°C, or gas mark 4) and lightly grease a 13 x 15-inch (33 x 38 cm) baking pan.

2. With a hand mixer or wooden spoon, blend the butter, brown sugar, and agave nectar. Beat in the eggs, one at a time with a hand mixer or a fork. Add the *Slow Cooker Steel-Cut Oats and Berries* and vanilla, mixing well.

3. In a separate bowl, combine the baking soda, sea salt, cinnamon, flaxseed, and flour.

4. Add the raisins to the flour mixture and coat well.

5. Add the raisin and flour mixture to the oatmeal mixture and stir to combine. Pour the batter into the prepared pan.

6. Bake for 20 to 25 minutes.

7. Top with fresh berries if desired.

Friends and Family Pizza

16+ months

YIELD: 6 TO 8 SERVINGS

Bringing friends and family together to make pizzas and have a fun picnic is a great way to enjoy a relaxed summer evening. What I love is that almost every age can enjoy playing with and rolling out dough, and you can individualize each pizza to fit picky tastes.

½ tablespoon (7 g) unsalted butter
1 red onion, sliced in big thin rounds
1 garlic clove, minced
2 packages premade pizza dough, organic if possible
1 cup (245 g) *Pizza Party Purée*, page 87
1 cup (150 g) grape tomatoes, halved and divided
1 cup (300 g) canned artichoke hearts, chopped and divided
2 cups (225 g) shredded mozzarella cheese, divided
1 cup (150 g) goat cheese, crumbled and divided
1 teaspoon fresh, chopped oregano, divided
1½ cup (60 g) fresh basil, chopped and divided

1. Preheat oven to 425°F (220°C, or gas mark 7), or an outside pizza brick oven to 500°F (250°C).

2. In a sauté pan, on medium heat, melt unsalted butter. Add red onions and garlic and sauté until browned and caramelized.

3. On a floured surface, roll out the dough into a thin sheet. Place the rolled out dough on a pizza stone or round baking sheet.

4. Spread the *Pizza Party Purée* on the pizzas as the sauce. Divide the sautéed red onions and garlic, grape tomatoes, artichoke hearts, mozzarella cheese, goat cheese, and fresh oregano and basil over both pizzas.

5. Cook for 12 to 15 minutes in a traditional oven, or 5 to 7 minutes in a heated outdoor brick oven.

Zesty Crab Cakes

15+ months

YIELD: 8 TO 10 PATTIES, OR SERVINGS

....

Crab cakes are the perfect food in my book! Try this with your favorite aioli or even just traditional tartar sauce and lemon!

1 cup (110 g) panko bread crumbs, divided
1 large egg, lightly beaten
2 tablespoons (28 ml) milk
1 teaspoon Worcestershire sauce
2 teaspoons spicy mustard
½ teaspoon Old Bay seasoning
1 teaspoon hot sauce
2 scallions, finely diced
2 tablespoons (28 ml) lemon juice
2 tablespoons (12 g) lemon zest
1 teaspoon sea salt
1 teaspoon pepper
¾ pound (340 g) lump crab, picked over
½ cup (125 g) Crab, Lemon, and Bell Pepper Textured Meal, page 88
1½ tablespoons (22 ml) coconut oil

1. In a small mixing bowl, combine ½ cup of the panko, egg, and milk and whisk together. Add all of the remaining ingredients, except the coconut oil and extra panko.

2. Shape into 8 to 10 patties, depending on size, keeping in mind that smaller crab cakes are better for smaller hands. Refrigerate for approximately 20 minutes, until firm.

3. Coat the cakes with the remaining panko.

4. Heat coconut oil in a sauté pan on medium heat. Cook patties 3 to 4 minutes per side, until crisp and golden brown. Serve warm.

Nectarine Teething Biscuits

12+ months

YIELD: 12 TO 15 TEETHING BISCUITS

....

Teething biscuits are awesome when baby starts cutting those first teeth, and this recipe is so tasty that you can call them cookies for your older toddlers and kids! Plus you won't have to buy the ready-made versions at the grocery store anymore!

1 egg, beaten
½ cup (125 g) Pure Nectarine Purée, page 89
2 tablespoons (40 g) raw agave nectar
¾ cup (100 g) whole wheat flour
1½ tablespoons (12 g) nonfat dry milk
1 tablespoon (8 g) coconut flour
1 tablespoon (8 g) ground flaxseed
1 tablespoon (8 g) chia seeds

1. Preheat the oven to 350°F (180°C, or gas mark 4).

2. In a medium bowl, stir together the egg, Pure Nectarine Purée, and agave nectar

3. In a separate bowl, combine the whole wheat flour, dry milk, coconut flour, flax, and chia seeds.

4. Stir the purée mixture into the dry ingredients until a smooth dough forms.

5. On a lightly floured surface, roll dough out to ¼-inch (6 mm)-thickness.

6. Cut into desired shapes and place onto parchment-lined baking sheet.

7. Bake for 15 minutes, until firm.

8. Cool and store in an airtight container at room temperature.

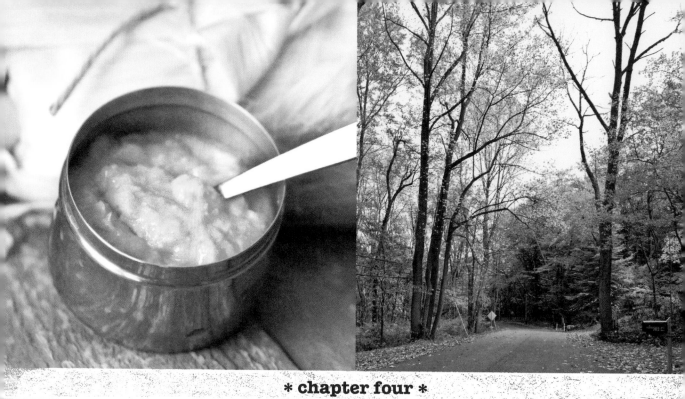

fall purées

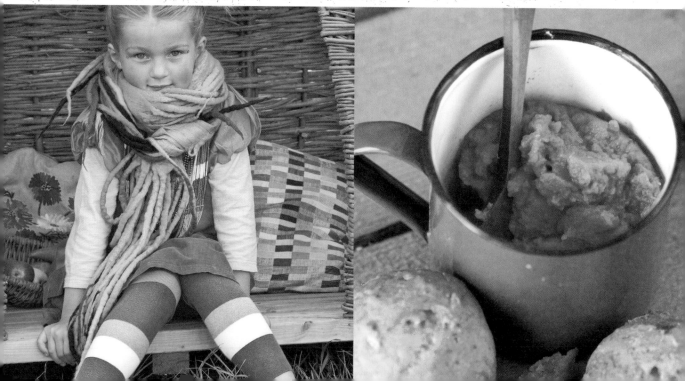

Welcome to fall, when the leaves turn gold, red, and orange, the winds get brisk, and you need to start bundling up. Babies just learning to walk stumble through big leafy piles, and kids are getting their last tree-swinging days in. The air is crisp, and the harvest of the season brings us foods that are meant to boost our immunity. Fall squashes, pumpkins, pomegranates, crisp apples, and tart cranberries all play a special role in feeding our bodies what they need during this bountiful season. If you have a baby lucky enough to start eating her first foods during the fall, then she will be blessed with fall flavors that are not only easily digestible, but naturally sweet and delicious. What I love about this season is the spirit of harvesting what we have grown both in our lives and in the ground, and bringing our loved ones together in the spirit of community and gratitude.

The Importance of Community

Food brings people together and your growing family can be a part of sharing goodness with each other, your friends, and your local community. Although we are the primary caregivers of our children, we need each other to help them grow and become diverse individuals in the world. We nurture them and keep them close, but need our village to help round out the edges and offer our children a bigger perspective of the world.

Nurturing a Family Community

Seeing your family as a community, where everyone needs to work together to make every day flow, is a great way to teach your children about the importance of sharing. Allow your older children to take on some responsibility to help with the younger ones from time to time. For example, I allow my daughter Lotus to help feed my little one River. He enjoys it, and she feels proud of her accomplishment in helping. I also expect all the children to bring the dishes over to the sink after dinner. Even the baby is capable of this task at 18 months.

Bringing Together Community with Food Swaps

Hosting a food swap is a simple way to bring together local communities, collect fresh homemade edibles, and never exchange a penny! Food swaps are where folks gather together in a home, community center, church, or school and exchange homemade culinary deliciousness. The only rules are that the edibles must be homegrown, homemade, or hand-foraged, and presented in reusable, earth-friendly packaging. These goodies become your own personal currency in swapping out items that you may want to snag. Contemporary swappers are fellow food-lovers, gardeners, home cooks, moms into organics, and super foodies who are offering up unique culinary creations in a friendly and fun exchange.

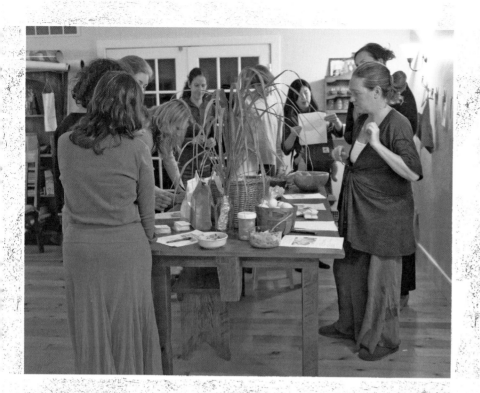
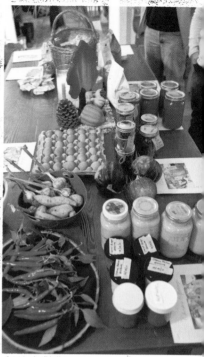

I recently hosted a food swap at my home, and the gathering attracted 25 local foodies. The food swag included delectables such as fresh duck eggs, homemade horseradish-infused vodka, freshly brewed concord grape soda, sweet potato maple butter, roasted garlic butter, homemade granola, sea salt caramel apples, elderberry syrup, jams, spreads, breads, fresh picked garlic, freshly milled flours, lemongrass, and cashew milks.

Food swaps are great for new moms because you can host a themed "baby food swap" where, for example, each of you commits to making ten jars of one purée from this book. The host invites at least 10 moms with their babies (so you are making friends and allowing your babies social play time) and each of you swap out jars with one another. When you leave, you should have ten varieties of homemade goodness ready and waiting for your baby to eat! It is an easy, fun, and cost-effective way to offer fresh, local, organic foods to your baby.

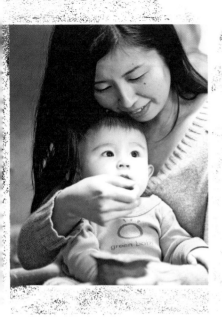
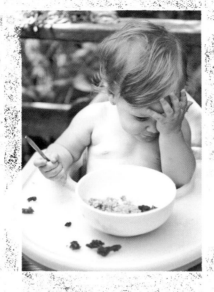
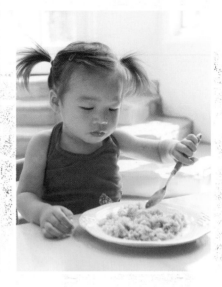

Understanding Baby's Cues

You may notice your baby eating greater and greater quantities of your deliciously prepared purées only to suddenly start refusing them all together. This is one sign that your baby is ready for more textured meals. Nobody can tell you exactly when this moment will come, which is why listening to your baby's cues is so important. Pay attention to his ability to handle little bites of texture so you will be able to gauge if he is ready for more texture and more food.

Keep in mind that some babies prefer purées for quite a while. If your child falls into that category, do not worry. He will like textured meals at some point; it just may take a little longer to get there. My daughter Lotus did not even start eating solids at all until she was about 11 months old. She simply was not interested. Then one day she did, and she went crazy for food. Today, at age 7, she is still an adventurous eater.

The one thing I want to reiterate is not to panic about food. Look closely at your own beliefs around food so you can feed your baby at his own pace and within the scope of his developing palate. Babies are excellent at reading our moods and can sense when we are worried. This tends to make the process of eating not fun for anyone. Just remember that every baby is as different as every adult, and we cannot say one thing works for all children. I can offer some guidance and say this is usually how it works, but nothing is absolute, which is why listening and paying close attention to your baby is the only sure way to make sure his specific needs are being met.

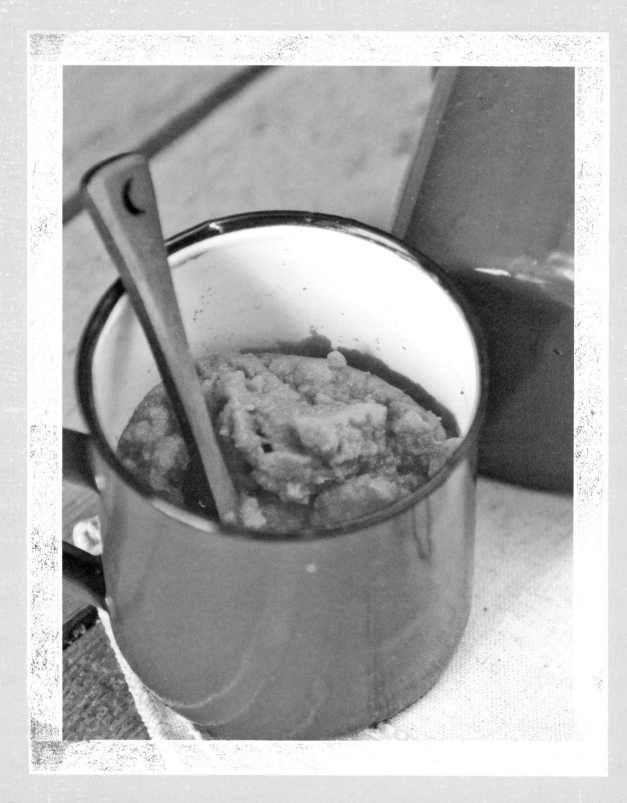

Apple, Squash, and Raisin Purée

7+ months

YIELD: 3 CUPS (750 G), OR 10 SERVINGS

2-IN-1 OPTION: **SPICED SQUASH AND APPLE MINI MUFFINS,** PAGE 130

....

Both apples and butternut squash are wonderful first foods for baby. They both are easily digestible, high in vitamins A and C, and offer a sweet flavor combination that babies love. Adding the raisins gives this recipe a special touch and an extra boost of fiber.

3 Fuji apples
½ butternut squash
¼ (35 g) cup raisins

1. Peel, core, and cut the apples into 1-inch (2.5 cm) pieces.

2. Peel and cube the butternut squash into 1-inch (2.5 cm) pieces.

3. Steam the apples and butternut squash together for 10 to 12 minutes, or until soft. Add the raisins and steam for 2 additional minutes. Reserve the liquid from the steamer.

4. Purée the apple, butternut squash, and raisins in a food processor with ½ cup (120 ml) of the reserved liquid. Add more liquid as needed to obtain the desired consistency.

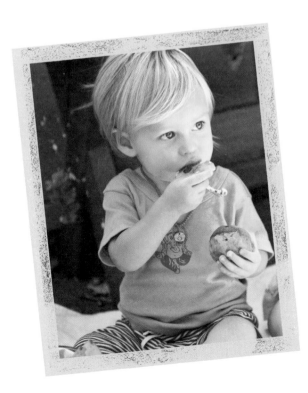

Red Lentil and Onion Textured Meal

9+ months

YIELD: 4 CUPS (1 KG), OR 10 BABY SERVINGS

2-IN-1 OPTION: **SPICY RED LENTIL SOUP,** PAGE 131

Lentils are full of fiber and taste delicious. I personally like how versatile they are and that you can turn this super protein into so many different meals. They are also another unique flavor profile that expands your baby's palate. This recipe is done in the slow cooker, and if you put it on before you go to bed, in the morning you will have a beautiful lentil dish that requires no further preparation.

2 cups (384 g) red lentils, uncooked
6 cups (1.5 L) vegetable broth
1 small onion, chopped
3 garlic cloves, chopped
1 teaspoon freshly grated ginger
1 teaspoon (fresh thyme)

1. In a slow cooker, combine all the ingredients and mix well.
2. Cook on low for 6 to 8 hours, until the mixture takes on a somewhat creamy texture.
3. Serve warm.

Pure Butternut Squash Purée

6+ months

YIELD: 4 TO 5 CUPS (1 TO 1.25 KG), OR 12 TO 15 BABY SERVINGS

2-IN-1 OPTION: **BUTTERNUT SQUASH MAC-N-CHEESE**, PAGE 132

Butternut squash is a butter flavored, easily digestible veggie that is high in vitamin C. It's the per-fect first food for your baby. One squash makes so much purée that there is always plenty left over to throw into cookies, breads, or in this case, mac-n-cheese.

1 butternut squash, cut in half

1. Preheat oven to 350°F (180°C, or gas mark 4).
2. Cut the butternut squash in half and scoop out the seeds.
3. On a lined parchment baking sheet, place the butternut squash halves face down. Bake for 40 minutes, or until soft.
4. Scoop the butternut squash from the skin and add to a blender with ½ cup (120 ml) water.
5. Add more water as needed to obtain the desired consistency.

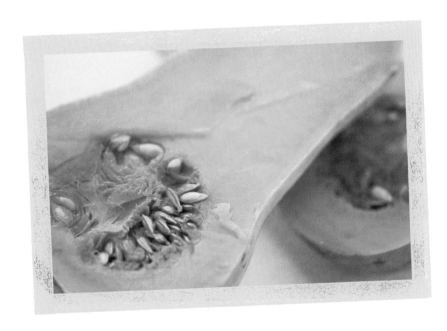

fall purées

Pure Pumpkin Raspberry Purée

8+ months

YIELD: 4 TO 5 CUPS (1 TO 1.25 KG), OR 12 TO 15 BABY SERVINGS

2-IN-1 OPTION: **WHOLE GRAIN PUMPKIN PANCAKES,** PAGE 133

Pumpkins are rich in vitamin A and fiber and can be used for many things during the fall. Most popular is the pumpkin pie of course, and while those are super tasty, there are a wide variety of uses for pumpkin. This is a great purée for baby because its nutty flavors and high nutritional content, but turn leftover purée into pancakes, and you have a winner for everyone.

1 small baking pumpkin, seeded
1 teaspoon olive oil
½ cup (120 ml) water
1 cup (125 g) fresh raspberries
1 banana

1. Preheat the oven to 350°F (180°C, or gas mark 4).
2. Cut the pumpkin in half and scoop out the seeds. Brush olive oil on the pumpkin flesh.
3. On a lined parchment baking sheet, place the pumpkins halves flesh side down on the sheet. Bake for 40 minutes, or until soft.
4. Scoop the pumpkin flesh from the skin and add to a blender with ½ cup (120 ml) water and raspberries.
5. Add banana to the blender and purée.
6. Add water as needed to obtain the desired consistency.

RECIPE NOTE

Make sure to save the pumpkin seeds for roasting!

fall purées

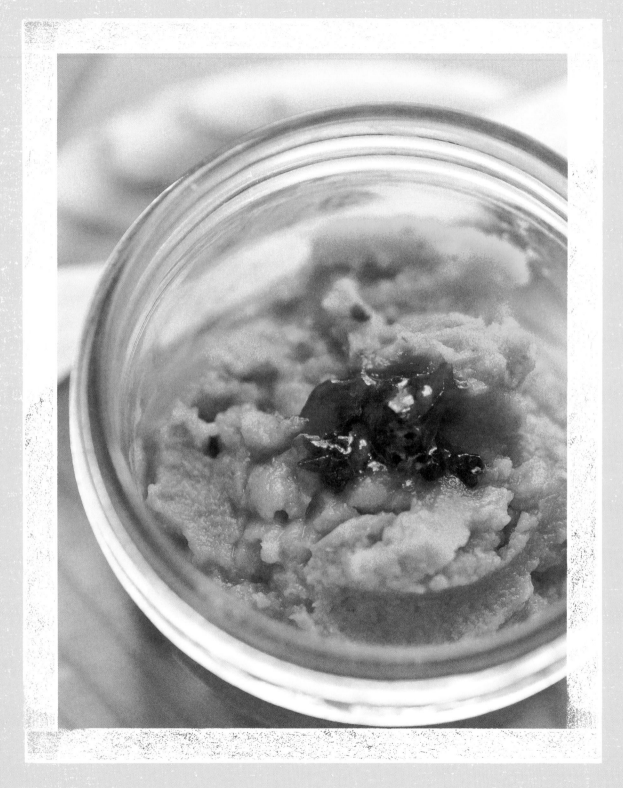

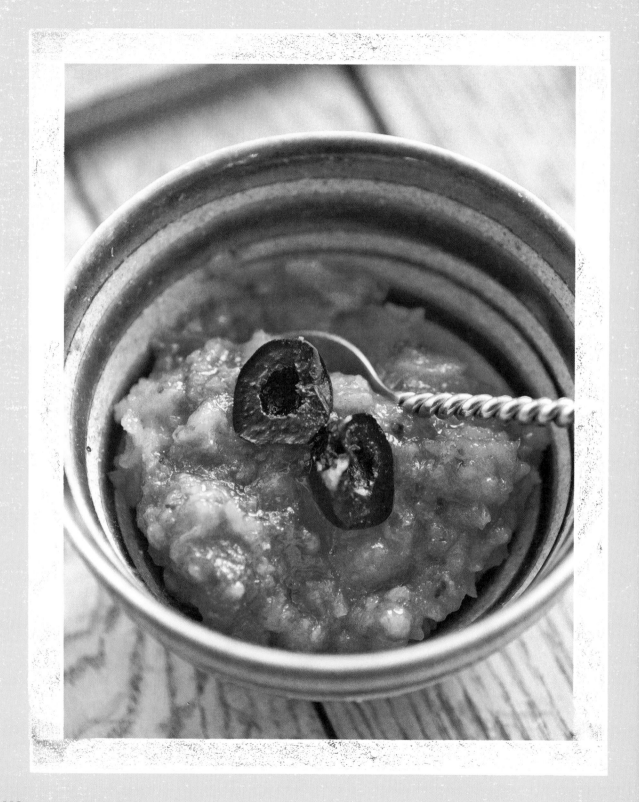

Cranberry, Apricot, and Sour Cherry Purée

8+ months

YIELD: 2 CUPS (500 G), OR 4 BABY SERVINGS

2-IN-1 OPTION: **FRUIT-FILLED PIE POPS,** PAGE 134

....

My oldest son and I love tart flavors. I think it's hereditary, and I find it so interesting that my other children have different sweet preferences. This particular purée is great as a pie pop filling, but it also makes a fantastic yogurt. Mix this with plain yogurt and you will have an amazingly creamy, sweet, and tart breakfast!

1 cup (100 g) fresh cranberries
3 apricots, chopped
1 cup (155 g) fresh or frozen sour cherries, pitted and chopped

1. Steam cranberries, apricots, and sour cherries together for 5 to 7 minutes, until they are soft.
2. Reserve the water from the steamer.
3. Blend the mixture in a blender until puréed. Add 1 teaspoon of reserved water at a time, if necessary, until desired consistency is achieved.

RECIPE NOTE

....

If you'd like your purée a little less tart, substitute the sour cherries with sweet and toss a few halves on top (assuming your baby can handle them).

fall purées

Acorn and Butternut Squash Purée

7+ months

YIELD: 4 TO 5 CUPS (1 TO 1.25 KG), OR 10 BABY SERVINGS

2-IN-1 OPTION: **SHEPHERD'S PIE,** PAGE 135

....

Squash season is always an amazing time of year. It's especially great for babies because these flavors are inviting, easily digestible, and tasty. One squash goes a long way, so this purée is great to use in other ways, which guarantees no waste. Note: Try to keep the skins intact if you are also making the Shepherd's Pie, as it's a fun way to serve the meal.

1 acorn squash
1 butternut squash

1. Preheat oven to 350°F (180°C, or gas mark 4).
2. Cut both squashes in half and scoop out the seeds.
3. On a lined parchment baking sheet, place the squash halves face down on the sheet and bake for 40 minutes, or until soft.
4. Scoop the squashes from the skins and add to a blender with ½ cup (120 ml) water.
5. Add more water as needed to obtain the desired consistency.

Why Eat Seasonally?

When you eat what is in season, you set your body up for good health. Mother Nature has a beautiful way of working in sync with us, as long as we pay attention and listen. Our bodies need and crave certain foods at different times of the year, and eating in this cyclical way brings a sense of reverence to our table. We gain respect for the seasons and how they change, and we honor our planet a little more.

For example, when it's hot in the summer, our bodies lose water. What is the most sought-after tasty summer treat? Chilled watermelon! This summer fruit is almost all water, so it naturally replenishes our depleted systems. In the fall and winter, we tend to get sick more often with colds and flus, and our bodies need more immune-building antioxidant foods, such as pomegranates and squash.

fall purées

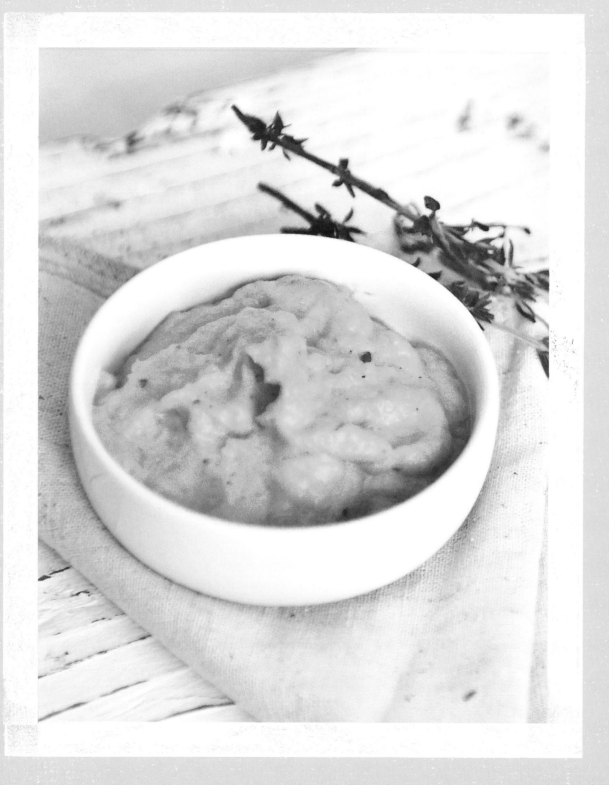

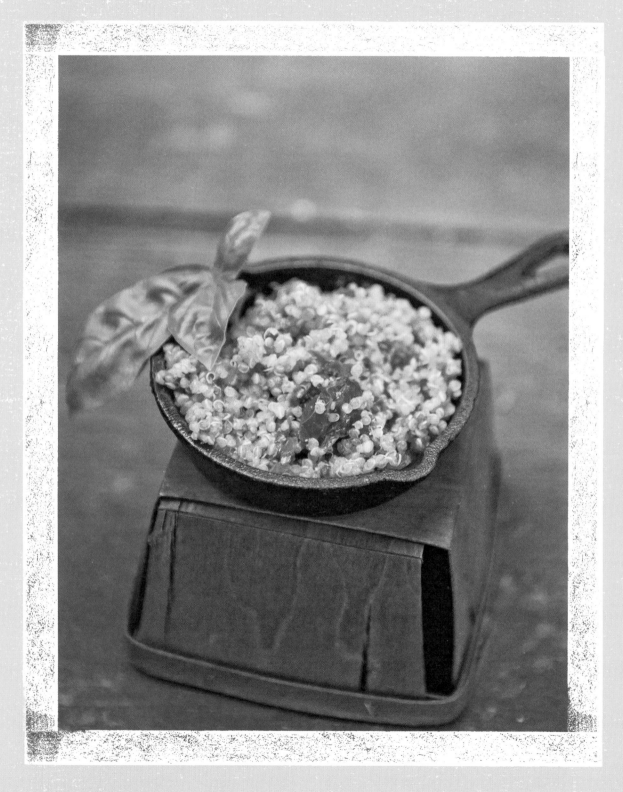

Sundried Tomato and Quinoa Textured Meal

11+ months

YIELD: 3 CUPS (750 G), OR 6 BABY SERVINGS

2-IN-1 OPTION: **SUNDRIED TOMATO AND FETA FLATBREAD PIZZA,** PAGE 136

Quinoa is one of the most nutritious super grains out there. It is high in protein, and its nutty flavor is delicious. What I love about quinoa is that you can adapt it to be sweet or savory, and either one is perfect. I even make a quinoa popsicle that babies love!

2 cups (350 g) quinoa, uncooked
2 cups (475 ml) water
2 cups (475 ml) vegetable broth
1 large garlic clove, minced
1 cup (145 g) chopped sundried tomatoes
4 fresh basil leaves, chopped small

1. In a medium pot, combine the quinoa, water, and vegetable broth and bring to a boil. Reduce to a simmer and let cook about 10 to 12 minutes, until the spiral-like germ uncoils from each grain.

2. While the quinoa is cooking, in a medium sauté pan, combine the garlic, sundried tomatoes, and basil. Sauté until garlic is browned and flavors meld together, about 5 minutes.

3. Combine the sundried tomato mixture with the quinoa and serve warm.

fall purées

Corn, Potato, and Carrot Purée

6+ months

YIELD: 4 CUPS (1 KG), OR 8 BABY SERVINGS

2-IN-1 OPTION: **SWEET CORN TAMALES**, PAGE 137

....

This is a simple flavored purée that is great for a new baby just trying out flavors because it's mild and sweet. If you make this dish when your corn is super fresh, then you grab that natural sweetness that Mother Nature provides. My babies always loved this combination.

4 yellow Finn potatoes, peeled and cubed
4 ears of fresh corn, shucked and kernels taken off the cob
2 carrots, peeled and chopped

1. Place potatoes and corn in a large pot of water and bring to a boil.
2. Let the potatoes and corn boil until soft, about 12 minutes.
3. While the corn and potatoes are boiling, steam the carrots for about 10 minutes, until soft.
4. Transfer the carrots and potato–corn mixture to a blender with a little reserved water from boiling the potatoes and corn or steaming the carrots. Blend to desired consistency.

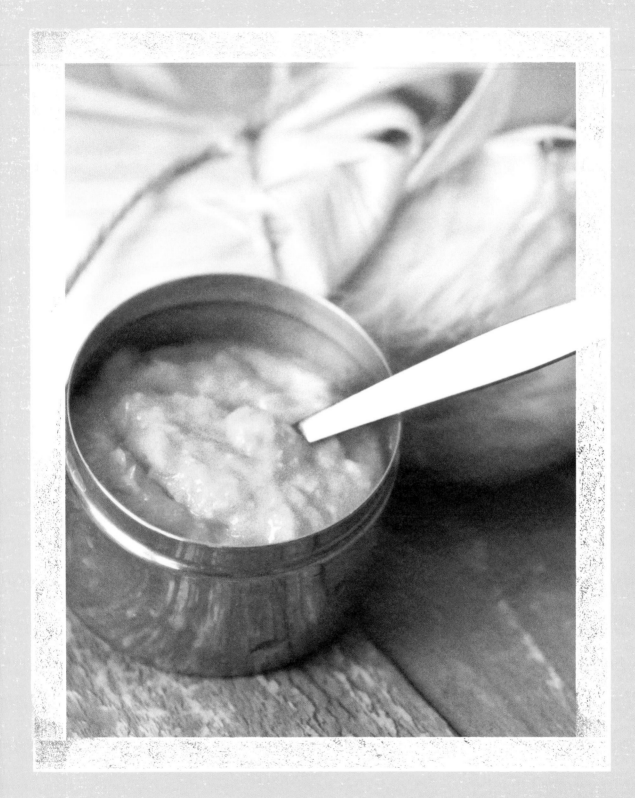

Sweet Potato and Banana Purée

6+ months

YIELD: 4 CUPS (1 KG), OR 12 BABY SERVINGS

2-IN-1 OPTION: **WHOLESOME RICE PUDDING,** PAGE 138

This combination is a wonderful first meal for your baby. Both sweet potatoes and bananas are low-allergen foods and easy for your baby to digest. They are also high in vitamin C and potassium.

1 sweet potato, peeled and diced
2 bananas, peeled and sliced

1. Steam the sweet potato for about 10 minutes or until soft. Reserve the liquid from the steamer.
2. Purée the sweet potato with the bananas in a food processor with ½ (120 ml) cup of the reserved liquid. Add more liquid as needed to obtain the desired consistency.

Baby Food Gardens

There is nothing like picking your own fruits and veggies from your own garden. If you plan ahead, you can create a garden that will produce foods that you can make baby food from. This is a great way to keep your food at its highest nutritional value as you basically just pick it and cook it! Some wonderful things to plant are sweet potatoes, onions, fall and winter squashes, berries, herbs, beans, peas, tomatoes, and carrots.

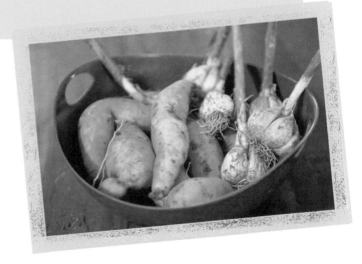

fall purées

Persimmon, Berry, and Mint Purée

10+ months

YIELD: 3 CUPS (750 G), OR 5 BABY SERVINGS

2-IN-1 OPTION: **PERSIMMON SOUFFLÉS,** PAGE 138

....

I love persimmons, and your baby is sure to love this combo! Persimmons are so pretty with their gorgeous orange skin, and they are the perfect combination of tart and sweet. They look somewhat like tomatoes. They are high in vitamin C and are a great source of fiber. I love to make recipe into a fall persimmon salad too, with just the fruit, mint, strawberries, and a little lemon juice. Yum!

3 persimmons, peeled chopped
2 cups (250 g) chopped strawberries or raspberries
¼ cup (24 g) chopped fresh mint

1. Steam persimmons for about 8 minutes until soft. Add the strawberries and steam for 2 more minutes. Reserve the water from the steamer.
2. Purée the mixture in a blender with the mint. Add 1 teaspoon (5 ml) of reserved water at a time, if necessary, until desired consistency is achieved.

RECIPE NOTE
....

The two most commonly available types of persimmons are Hachiya and Fuyu. Hachiya persimmons are larger and should not be eaten until very ripe (soft to the touch and almost to the point of mushy). Fuyu persimmons are smaller and more tomato-shaped, and may be eaten while still a bit firm.

Savory Carrot Purée

10+ months

YIELD: 3 CUPS (750 G), OR 10 BABY SERVINGS

2-IN-1 OPTION: **ROASTED DOUBLE CARROT SOUP,** PAGE 139

Carrots are sweet and delicious and make a wonderful meal for your baby. I like to add in a little flavor to boost the appeal. Turning this meal into a warm and inviting soup for the rest of your family is the perfect way to usher in the fall.

4 full carrots, peeled and diced
1 garlic clove, minced
1 tomato, chopped

1. Steam the carrots and garlic for about 10 minutes or until soft. Reserve the liquid from the steamer.

2. Add the tomato during the last two minutes.

3. Purée the carrot mixture in a food processor with ½ cup (120 ml) of the reserved liquid. Add more liquid as needed to obtain the desired consistency.

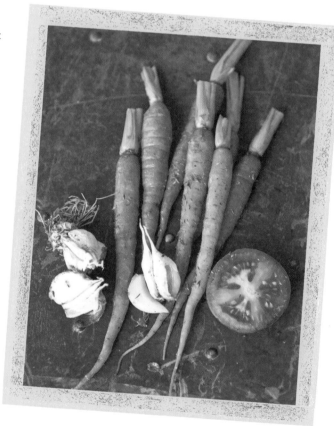

Pure Carrot Purée

7+ months

YIELD: 3 CUPS (750 G), OR 9 BABY SERVINGS

2-IN-1 OPTION: **MOIST AND HEARTY CARROT CAKE,** PAGE 140

....

The primary thing to keep in mind when feeding your baby carrots are the nitrate levels. Nitrates are naturally occurring elements in soil, but when commercial fertilizers are used, they can cause an excess of nitrates to build up in the soil (and surrounding well water) and leech into the plants. Because it's important that young babies not ingest high levels of nitrates, be sure to buy organic carrots or grow your own—particularly if you know your soil is safe.

6 large carrots, peeled and diced

1. Steam the carrots for about 10 minutes or until soft. Reserve the liquid from the steamer.
2. Purée the carrot in a food processor with ½ cup (120 ml) of the reserved liquid. Add more liquid as needed to obtain the desired consistency.

fall purées

Spinach, Kale, and Carrot Purée

7+ months

YIELD: 3 CUPS (750 G), OR 9 BABY SERVINGS

2-IN-1 OPTION: **EASY ENCHILADA BAKE,** PAGE 140

Getting your babies and children to eat greens is critical to their overall health. If you start early, you will be happier that your baby got used to the taste of succulent greens right out of the gate. My mama always said it's far easier to make knots than undo them. Starting off with healthy food is far easier than starting off with processed foods and then trying to go back in time. Start early and everyone is happy!

1 cup (30 g) spinach leaves, packed, stems removed
1 cup (30 g) kale leaves, chopped and packed, stems removed
3 large carrots, peeled and diced

1. Steam spinach and kale together for 3 to 5 minutes, until they are soft.
2. Set spinach and kale aside and steam the carrots for 8 to 9 minutes. You can do this simultaneously if you have 2 steamers. Reserve the water from the steamer.
3. Blend the spinach, kale, and carrot mixture in a blender until puréed. Add 1 teaspoon of reserved water at a time, if necessary, until desired consistency is achieved.

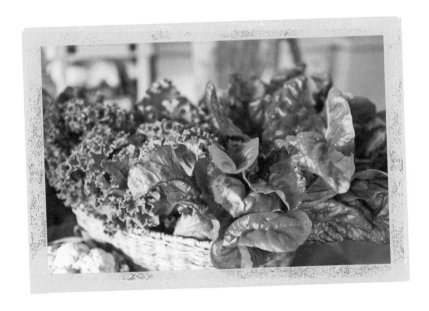

Pure Fuji Apple Purée

6+ months

YIELD: 3 CUPS (750 G), OR 10 BABY SERVINGS

2-IN-1 OPTION: **OATMEAL APPLE COOKIES,** PAGE 141

....

Apples are one of the best foods for all people; babies, kids, and adults. No matter how you eat it, an apple a day is a good way to keep illness away! Babies love this nature's treat and it is a wonderful first food, as this purée is easy on a delicate digestive system. Applesauce is one of the few purées that transcends the lines of baby/adult food. I still love eating homemade applesauce and find that it brings back amazing memories of my childhood with every bite.

4 Fuji apples, peeled and diced

1. Peel, core, and cut the apples into 1-inch (2.5 cm) pieces.
2. Steam the apples for about 10 minutes or until soft. Reserve the liquid from the steamer.
3. Purée the apple in a food processor or blender with ½ cup (120 ml) of the reserved liquid. Add more liquid as needed to obtain the desired consistency.

Make a Compost Bin!

Composting is the simple act of feeding the earth organic matter that can be naturally broken down and turned back into delicious fertilizer. Composting is great to teach your children and can be really simple. You can put all the food scraps in a composting bucket in the kitchen and have an older child take it out to the compost bin outside. Composting bins can be bought at your local hardware store or easily made at home. If you do not have older children, try taking on this job yourself to get into the habit now so you can try to teach your children about this practice as they grow. Remember that putting all of these practices into action will teach your child a healthy respect and reverence for the Earth and its natural resources and will empower them to understand more about where their food comes from and how the cycle of growing and recycling really works.

fall purées

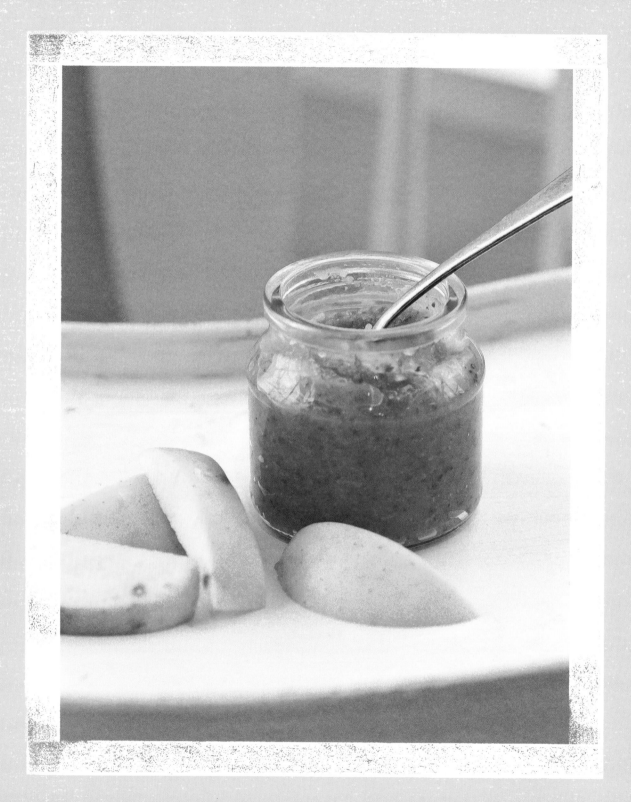

Spiced Apple, Pear, and Raisin Purée

8+ months

YIELD: 3 CUPS (750 G), OR 9 BABY SERVINGS
2-IN-1 OPTION: **FRUITY BREAD PUDDING,** PAGE 142

....

This is a lovely spiced-up version of an old classic that even adults will enjoy as a side dish. I love these flavors together, and if you can get your older kids out on an apple-picking adventure, you will have the freshest purée in town. If not, hit your local farmer's market to get these seasonal goodies.

3 Fuji apples, peeled and cubed
3 Bartlett pears, peeled and cubed
1 teaspoon cinnamon
½ cup (75 g) raisins

1. Peel, core, and cut the apples and pears into 1-inch (2.5 cm) pieces.
2. Sprinkle cinnamon overs the apples and pears and steam for 8 to 10 minutes, or until soft.
3. Add in the raisins and steam for 2 additional minutes. Reserve the liquid from the steamer.
4. Purée the apple, pears, and raisins in a food processor with ½ cup (120 ml) of the reserved liquid. Add more liquid as needed to obtain the desired consistency.

fall purées

Baby Refried Beans and Cheese

11+ months

YIELD: 5 CUPS (1.25 KG), OR 15 BABY SERVINGS

2-IN-1 OPTION: **CRISPY BAKED TAQUITOS,** PAGE 143

....

Beans are packed with protein and essential for babies who do not prefer meat, or if you choose to raise your baby vegetarian or vegan. Adding onions and herbs give the beans flavor and make for a nice comforting lunch or snack throughout the day.

2 cups (500 g) dried pinto beans, washed and soaked overnight

4 cups (950 ml) water

4 cups (950 ml) vegetable or chicken stock

1 bay leaf

1 onion, peeled and finely chopped

2 cloves of garlic, chopped

2 teaspoons (10 ml) coconut oil (or your preferred cooking oil)

½ cup (75 g) grated cheddar cheese (leave out if vegan)

1. Place beans, water, stock, bay leaf, onion, and garlic in a large cooking pot.

2. Cover and bring to a boil.

3. Reduce to low heat and let simmer for 1½ hours, or until beans are tender.

4. Remove bay leaf and drain bean mixture, reserving broth in another pot or bowl.

5. In a large nonstick pan on medium heat, add coconut oil and then add in bean mixture with 1 cup of the broth. Reserve remaining broth for another use.

6. Cook the beans, stirring frequently and mashing as you stir to reach the consistency your baby prefers. Continue adding in water as needed to get the beans to a nice thick paste and not dry.

7. Add in the cheese and allow to melt into the beans. Serve warm.

fall purées

Ginger-Spiced Pumpkin Purée

10+ months

YIELD: 4 TO 5 CUPS (1 TO 1.25 KG), OR 10 BABY SERVINGS

2-IN-1 OPTION: **APPLE PUMPKIN BUTTER,** PAGE 143

Pumpkin is so nutritionally packed with vitamins that getting babies hooked on it is a great accomplishment—and an easy thing to do when you blend it with a little spice. So many pumpkins go to waste during the fall because folks don't think to cook them up, but you should! Use as many as you can when they are ripe and at their best, and don't throw away those seeds either. Roast them with lime juice and salt for a snack, or let older kids watercolor paint them and string them into necklaces!

1 small baking pumpkin
1 teaspoon (5 ml) olive oil
½ cup (120 ml) water
1 teaspoon ground ginger
½ teaspoon cinnamon
½ teaspoon ground nutmeg

1. Preheat the oven to 350°F (180°C).
2. Cut the pumpkin in half and scoop out the seeds. (Make sure to save the seeds for roasting.) Brush olive oil on the pumpkin flesh.
3. On a baking sheet lined with parchment, place the pumpkins halves flesh side down. Bake for 40 minutes, or until soft.
4. When cool enough to handle, scoop the pumpkin flesh from the skin and add to a blender with water and spices.
5. Purée until smooth. Add water as needed to obtain the desired consistency.

fall purées

Spiced Squash and Apple Mini Muffins

12+ months

YIELD: 20 TO 25 MINI MUFFINS, OR SERVINGS

These muffins are perfect for toddlers' little hands and are packed with the same goodness they got when they were babies. These are also a great cupcake alternative for a one-year-old's birthday party or as a midday snack.

2 cups (250 g) whole wheat pastry flour
1 teaspoon baking soda
2 teaspoons (5 g) cinnamon
1 teaspoon fresh nutmeg
¼ teaspoon ground cloves
¼ teaspoon allspice
½ teaspoon sea salt
1 cup (340 g) raw agave nectar
½ cup (112 g) unsalted butter, softened
3 eggs
1½ cups (370 g) Apple, Squash, and Raisin Purée, page 107
Fresh butter, fruit, and raisins, for serving

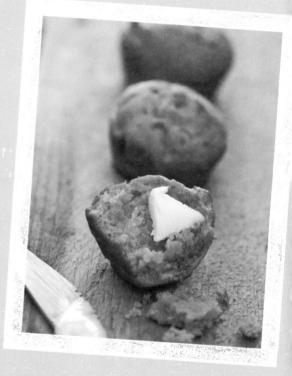

1. Preheat the oven to 350°F (180°C, or gas mark 4).
2. Combine all dry ingredients.
3. In a separate bowl, using either a hand-held or stand mixer on medium speed, beat butter with the agave nectar.
4. Beat in the eggs, one at a time.
5. Add in the *Apple, Squash, and Raisin Purée.*
6. On low speed, add the flour mixture a little bit at a time until you have added it all and you have a cake-like batter.
7. Line a mini muffin pan with cupcake liners and distribute batter equally, filling each about three-quarters full.
8. Cook for 18 to 20 minutes, or until a toothpick inserted in the center comes out clean.
9. Serve warm with fresh butter, fruit, and raisins, if desired.

Spicy Red Lentil Soup

12+ months

SERVES: 8 CUPS (2 KG), OR 6 ADULT SERVINGS, OR 10 KID SERVINGS

In the fall, I always have a soup on the stove when my kids come home from school. This is a wonderful warm and filling after school snack, and I find that it feeds a lot of people for not a lot of money. My kids always have their friends over for play dates, and a nice warm soup is the perfect way to feed everyone. Throw in some rustic style garlic bread, and you have a very satisfying meal.

1 tablespoon (14 g) unsalted butter
1 large yellow onion, chopped
1 teaspoon sea salt
1 to 2 teaspoons pepper
6 cups (1.5 L) water
2 cups (490 g) *Red Lentil and Onion Textured Meal*, page 108
¼ teaspoon ground cloves
1 teaspoon Chinese five-spice powder
½ teaspoon ground cumin
2 vegetable bouillon cubes
2 large whole tomatoes, chopped
3 carrots, cut into rounds or diced
1 long celery rib, diced
3 limes, cut into wedges, for serving

1. In a large soup pot, melt the butter and sauté the chopped onion until browned.
2. Season with salt and pepper.
3. Add the water and the *Red Lentil and Onion Textured Meal* for Baby to the pot.
4. Add the cloves, five spice, cumin, and bouillon cubes and stir the soup well.
5. Add tomatoes, carrots, and celery, and let soup simmer for 10 to 12 minutes until all the flavors meld together. Add in a touch more salt or pepper to taste.
6. Squeeze lime wedge on top just before serving.

RECIPE NOTE

Chinese five-spice powder is a mix of fennel, cloves, cinnamon, star anise and Szechuan peppercorns. It is said to encompass all five flavors—sweet, sour, bitter, pungent, and salty—and adds a great kick to soups, marinades, and more. Find it at any well-stocked grocery or Asian market.

Butternut Squash Mac-n-Cheese

15+ months

YIELD: 10 SERVINGS

Mac-n-cheese is a kid's classic. Add the butternut squash, and it raises the nutritional level and flavor. I like this recipe because it's a healthier than the traditional version and my kids love it!

6 cups (1.5 L) water
2 cups (210 g) macaroni noodles, uncooked
¼ cup (60 ml) heavy cream
1 teaspoon nutmeg
1 cup (120 g) shredded cheddar cheese
¼ teaspoon sea salt
Pepper to taste
1 cup (245 g) *Pure Butternut Squash Purée*, page 109
½ cup (60 g) panko bread crumbs

1. Preheat oven to 350°F (180°C, or gas mark 4)
2. In a large pot, boil the water. Add the macaroni noodles and boil for 8 minutes. Drain.
3. In a separate pot on medium heat, mix cream, nutmeg, cheese, salt, and pepper. Heat until cheese melts.
4. Add the *Pure Butternut Squash Purée* and cooked noodles, and stir to combine.
5. Pour mixture in a baking dish and top with panko bread crumbs.
6. Bake for 20 to 25 minutes.

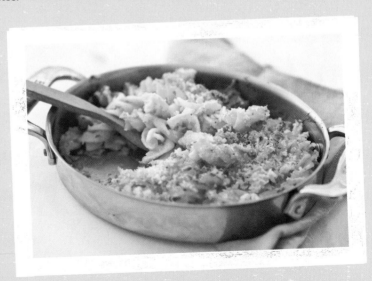

Whole Grain Pumpkin Pancakes

15+ months

YIELD: 12 TO 15 MEDIUM-SIZE PANCAKES

Pancakes are warm are comforting in this cool fall season, and there is just something fun about gathering around a table to share this traditional breakfast. Pumpkin spice gives the perfect fall complement to this meal and steps up the healthful component as well.

2 cups (250 g) whole wheat pastry flour
¼ teaspoon sea salt
1½ teaspoons ground cinnamon
½ teaspoon ground nutmeg
½ teaspoon allspice
½ teaspoon ground ginger
1 teaspoon baking soda
1½ teaspoons (7 g) baking powder
1 cup (235 ml) milk
1½ cups (370 g) *Pure Pumpkin Raspberry Purée*, page 110
1 teaspoon vanilla extract
2 eggs
1 tablespoon (14 g) unsalted butter
Pure maple syrup, for serving

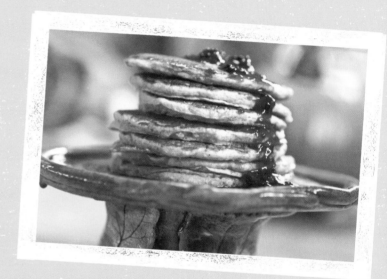

1. In a large mixing bowl, combine flour, salt, cinnamon, nutmeg, allspice, ginger, baking soda, and baking powder.

2. In a separate bowl, combine milk, *Pure Pumpkin Raspberry Purée*, vanilla, and eggs.

3. Add wet ingredients to dry ingredients and mix until combined.

4. Melt about 1 tablespoon (14 g) of butter in a large skillet or griddle and heat to medium-high. Ladle pancake batter into skillet to make medium sized pancakes. As soon as bubbles begin to form on the top side of the pancakes, flip. Both sides should be lightly browned when done.

5. Remove pancakes from skillet and serve immediately with maple syrup.

RECIPE NOTE

Take your maple syrup over the top by simmering a cup or so (340 g) in a saucepan with a couple generous handfuls of either blackberries, blueberries, or raspberries (or all 3)! Let cook until the berries break down and can be mashed with the back of a spoon. Serve warm over pancakes.

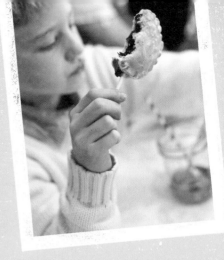

Fruit-Filled Pie Pops

15+ months

YIELD: 15 TO 18 PIE POPS

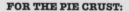

These pie pops are the cutest food ever! It really does not get better than pie on a stick.

FOR THE PIE CRUST:

1⅓ cup (166 g) all-purpose unbleached flour

½ teaspoon natural cane sugar, such as Sucanat

¼ teaspoon salt

1 stick (½ cup or 112 g) unsalted butter, cut into 1-inch (2.5 cm) pieces

½ cup (120 ml) ice cold water

1 to 2 eggs, lightly beaten, for brushing on pie pops

FOR THE FILLING:

2 cups (500 g) *Cranberry, Apricot, and Sour Cherry Purée*, page 113

2 tablespoons arrowroot powder

3 tablespoons (60 g) honey

Egg wash, for brushing

1. Preheat oven to 350°F (180°C, or gas mark 4).

2. Combine flour, sugar, and salt in the bowl of your stand mixer and lightly combine.

3. Turn mixer on low to medium speed. Drop in the butter pieces one at a time and mix until mixture resembles coarse meal, with pea-size pieces of butter. Slowly add in water until a smooth dough forms (you should still be able to see bits of butter in the dough). If the dough is still too dry, add water by the teaspoon until it comes together.

4. Use your hands to shape the dough into a nice ball. No need to refrigerate dough before using.

5. Roll out dough onto a floured surface, about ¼-inch (6 mm)-thick. Poke the rolled out crust a few times with a fork. Using a round cookie cutter or other 4- to 5-inch (10 to 13 cm)-diameter cutter, cut out 30 to 36 circles, rerolling as necessary.

6. Place half of the circles on a baking sheet (or two), leaving space in between for the sticks.

7. In a large bowl, combine *Cranberry, Apricot, and Sour Cherry Purée*, arrowroot, and honey, stirring well. Place a small spoonful of filling directly in the middle of the dough circles on the baking sheet(s). Place pop stick on top of the filling and press it down into the dough. Place each remaining dough round on top of each filled round, pressing edges together gently with wet fingers. Press around the edges of each pie pop with a fork to seal and crimp.

8. Make a small slit on the top of each pie pop with a knife, being careful not to slice all the way through the dough. Brush the top of each pop with the egg wash.

9. Bake pie pops on a parchment-lined baking sheet for about 15 minutes, until golden brown.

Shepherd's Pie

15+ months

YIELD: 4 TO 5 SERVINGS

Shepherd's Pie is a classic dish that everyone in my house loves. This little twist leaves out the meat and swaps traditional mashed potatoes for squash, giving the dish a whole new depth of flavor, along with some additional nutritional value. For a purely vegetarian version, swap out the chicken broth for vegetable broth.

1 tablespoon (14 g) unsalted butter

2 tablespoons (28 ml) Bragg Liquid Aminos

2 tablespoons (28 ml) low-sodium soy sauce

1 large yellow onion, diced small

½ cup (65 g) diced carrots

½ cup (100 g) chopped celery

1 cup (150 g) peas, shelled
(fresh or frozen works well)

1 tablespoon fresh chopped rosemary

½ tablespoon fresh chopped thyme

2 garlic cloves, minced

4 cups (1 L) chicken broth

¼ teaspoon sea salt

Pepper to taste

½ cup (58 g) shredded cheddar cheese

4 cups (980 g) *Acorn and Butternut Squash Purée*, page 114

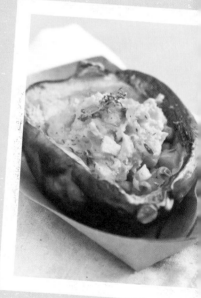

1. In a large saucepan over medium-high heat, melt the butter. Add the liquid aminos and soy sauce.

2. Add the onions, carrots, celery, peas, rosemary, thyme, and garlic and sauté for 5 to 7 minutes.

3. Add broth, salt, and pepper and bring to a boil. Turn off heat and set aside.

4. Preheat the oven to broil.

5. Combine the cheese and *Acorn and Butternut Squash Purée* in a bowl and set aside.

6. Scoop some of the veggie mixture into 4 individual pie tins or ramekins, or into the scooped-out acorn squash shells (if you still have them), making sure to get a little broth and mostly veggies into each one. Top with *Acorn and Butternut Squash Purée* mixture.

7. Place the tins on a baking sheet and put under the broiler for 3 to 4 minutes or until browned on top. Serve warm.

RECIPE NOTES

> If you don't have individual pie tins, just use a regular, oven-safe baking dish.

> Bragg Liquid Aminos is a natural liquid protein concentrate, derived from soybeans. It contains important healthy amino acids and protein and is a great addition to veggies, grains, meat dishes, and more.

Sundried Tomato and Feta Flatbread Pizza

18+ months

YIELD: 4 ADULT SERVINGS, OR 6 KID SERVINGS

I love these pizzas because they are tasty and easy to make, not to mention wonderfully nutritious and packed with flavor. They are fun to make for a lunch with friends with kids, as they can feed a lot of folks in a simple, quick way.

3 pieces of garlic flatbread
2 cups (490 g) *Sundried Tomato and Quinoa Textured Meal*, page 117
1 cup (150 g) feta cheese, divided among 3 flatbreads
1 red onion, sliced in thin rounds
½ cup (20 g) fresh basil leaves, chopped

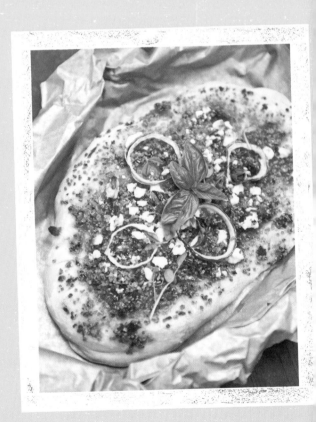

1. Preheat oven to 425°F (220°C, or gas mark 7).

2. Place flatbreads in the oven on a pizza stone or a cookie sheet, without any of the toppings, and bake for 5 minutes.

3. Remove the flatbread from the oven and spread *Sundried Tomato and Quinoa Textured Meal* for Baby over the top.

4. Add feta cheese, red onion slices, and basil.

5. Bake flatbreads for 10 to 12 more minutes, until slightly browned.

Sweet Corn Tamales

16+ months

YIELD: 15 TO 20 TAMALES, OR SERVINGS

Tamales are a traditional Mexican dish that really celebrates the culture. The sweet corn version is fun to make and presents another great opportunity to include your kids in the process. You will need cornhusks, masa (prepared corn dough found at a Mexican food store), and a little bit more time than usual for this recipe. This is a good recipe to make on the weekend when you may have a little more leisure time to spare.

3 cups (750 g) *Corn, Potato, and Carrot Purée*, page 118
½ (170 g) cup honey
2 pounds (907 g) prepared masa
20 dried corn husks, soaked in warm water until pliable (about 20 minutes)
½ cup (8 g) fresh chopped cilantro
1 cup (230 g) sour cream, to garnish

1. Mix the *Corn, Potato, and Carrot Purée* with the honey.

2. Mix the masa by hand with purée mixture.

3. Scoop 3 to 4 tablespoons of mixture onto the center of the smooth side of each corn husk. Fold sides and bottom in and either tie off or leave folded.

4. Cook tamales in your steamer by lining the basket with any extra corn husks and stacking them on top of each other. Make sure that your tamales do not touch the water.

5. Steam for 45 to 65 minutes, until the masa no longer sticks to the corn husk.

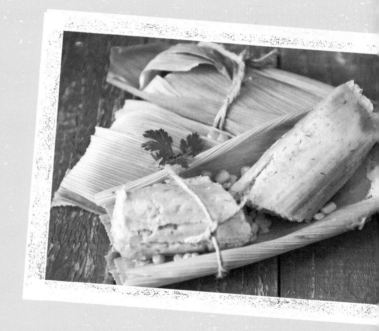

Wholesome Rice Pudding

15+ months

YIELD: 4 CUPS (1 KG), OR 6 TO 8 SERVINGS

Rice is a sacred food around the world and a major staple for many cultures. Rice pudding is a sweet treat that everyone loves and is easy to make. This is a filling dessert that has a healthier twist than most.

2 cups (475 ml) water
1 cup (195 g) basmati rice, uncooked
3 cups (709 ml) whole milk
1 cup (245 g) Sweet Potato and Banana Purée, page 120
1 cup (235 g) whipping cream
¼ teaspoon cinnamon
¼ teaspoon allspice
¼ teaspoon nutmeg
½ cup (170 g) raw agave nectar

1. In a medium saucepan, boil water and rice together, covered. After the rice comes to a boil, reduce to simmer and cook for 12 to 15 minutes, stirring once or twice.

2. Add the rest of the ingredients and bring back to a boil. Reduce back to a simmer and cook for 25 to 30 minutes, uncovered. Keep stirring so the rice pudding does not burn.

3. When rice has reached a thick, creamy consistency, remove from heat.

4. Serve warm.

Persimmon Soufflés

16+ months

YIELD: 6 SERVINGS

Soufflés are so delicate and delicious, and this fall version is a wonderful treat for after dinner on a special occasion. My son Zoe, who wants to be a chef, loves soufflés and anything tart, so this is one I like to make him on his birthday, given he was born in autumn.

2 cups Persimmon, Berry, and Mint Purée, page 121
½ cup (85 g) chopped strawberries
Zest and juice of 1 lemon
1 cup (235 ml) whole milk
1 tablespoon (6 g) arrowroot
1 cup (200 g) pure cane sugar, divided
3 large eggs, separated
1 tablespoon (14 g) unsalted butter

1. Preheat oven to 400°F (200°C, or gas mark 6). Coat six small ramekins with butter.

2. Place about a tablespoon of the Persimmon, Berry, and Mint Purée and a few small strawberry pieces into each ramekin.

3. In a medium saucepan over medium heat, combine lemon zest and juice, milk, arrowroot, ½ cup sugar, and the egg yolks and bring to a boil. Whisk constantly until a pudding consistency forms, then whisk in butter until melted. Transfer to a mixing bowl.

4. In a separate bowl, with a hand mixer, beat the egg whites until soft peaks form, adding the remaining ½ cup (100 g) sugar toward the end. Carefully fold the whites into the pudding mixture.

5. Spoon the mixture over top of the berries in each ramekin. Bake for about 15 minutes, until it puffs up and is lightly golden.

Roasted Double Carrot Soup

12+ months

YIELD: 8 CUPS (2 KG), OR 10 TO 12 SERVINGS

....

When the fall rolls into our countryside, it gets cold, and my kids love warm food. This rustic soup is the perfect healthy fall evening meal and fills the house with a comforting smell that is so inviting it's likely to become a family favorite.

8 large carrots, peeled and sliced

6 garlic cloves, peeled

3 tablespoons (45 ml) olive oil

1 tablespoon (14 g) unsalted butter

1 large yellow onion, chopped

2 pinches sea salt

4 pinches pepper

1 teaspoon dried basil

4 cups (940 ml) chicken stock

2 vegetable bouillon cubes

2 cups (475 ml) water

2 cups (490 g) *Savory Carrot Purée*, page 122

1 pinch red pepper flakes

1. Preheat oven to 300°F (150°C, or gas mark 2).

2. Wash carrots and slice in half.

3. Place carrots and garlic on a parchment-lined baking sheet and lightly drizzle with olive oil. Roast for 45 minutes.

4. After the carrots have been cooking for 30 minutes, in a large soup pot, melt the butter and sauté the chopped onion until browned. Season with salt, pepper, and dried basil.

5. Add the roasted carrots and garlic to the pot.

6. Add chicken stock, bouillons cubes, water, *Savory Carrot Purée*, and red pepper flakes and let simmer for about 5 minutes.

7. Using a hand mixer or blender, purée soup until it is a smooth consistency.

Moist and Hearty Carrot Cake

12+ months

YIELD: 10 TO 12 SERVINGS

....

This is my all time, hands down, favorite dessert in the world. You absolutely must top it with either fresh whipped cream or cream cheese frosting! Yum!

2 cups (250 g) all-purpose flour
2 teaspoons (9 g) baking powder
1 teaspoon baking soda
1 teaspoon salt
2 teaspoons (5 g) ground cinnamon
¼ teaspoon nutmeg
¼ teaspoon allspice
¼ teaspoon ground ginger
2 cups (500 g) *Pure Carrot Purée*, page 123
1 cup (340 g) honey
1 cup (200 g) pure cane sugar
1½ cups (354 ml) sunflower oil
4 eggs
Freshly whipped cream or cream cheese frosting, optional

1. Preheat oven to 325°F (170° C). Grease and flour a 9 x 13-inch (23 x 33 cm) pan.

2. In a medium sized bowl, mix the flour, baking powder, baking soda, salt, and spices. Set aside.

3. In a large bowl, mix *Pure Carrot Purée*, honey, sugar, oil, and eggs.

4. Beat in flour mixture a little bit at a time, until there are no visible streaks of flour. Be careful not to overmix.

5. Pour mixture into prepared pan and bake for 35 to 40 minutes, or until a toothpick inserted into the center of the cake comes out clean. Allow to cool.

6. Top with fresh whipped cream or your favorite cream cheese frosting, if desired.

Easy Enchilada Bake

15+ months

YIELD: 6 SERVINGS

....

My kids love enchiladas, and this homey version is a rustic meal like mom would make. What is it about food that brings people together? I have often pondered this question, and I really think that it is the memories that a great meal produces that connects us and warms our homes and tummies.

1 tablespoon (15 ml) coconut oil
1 whole yellow onion, diced and sautéed
2 garlic cloves, minced
2½ cups (600 g) *Spinach, Kale, and Carrot Purée*, page 124
1 package of corn tortillas, divided
2 cups (750 g) organic whole black beans (canned is fine)
2 cups (225 g) shredded cheddar cheese
1 cup (230 g) sour cream, for serving

1. Preheat the oven to 350°F (180°C, or gas mark 4).

2. In a sauté pan, sauté the onion and garlic in coconut oil until caramelized and browned.

3. Mix the *Spinach, Kale, and Carrot Purée* with the onions and garlic.

4. In a glass baking dish, place a layer of corn tortillas, overlapping where needed.

5. Top the tortillas with the *Spinach, Kale, and Carrot Purée*.

6. Add a layer of black beans followed by a layer of cheese.

7. Repeat this process two more times and end with a layer of cheese.

8. Bake for 20 to 25 minutes and serve with sour cream.

Oatmeal Apple Cookies

12+ months

YIELD: 25 COOKIES, OR SERVINGS

Oatmeal cookies are my number one favorite cookie. My mom had a friend who baked the best oatmeal cookies, and right after I had my first son 14 years ago, she brought me over a tin full of these cookies. During my first days of breastfeeding my infant, I think I lived on them. (No wonder my teenager loves cookies so much!) I asked my mom to ask her friend what her secret ingredient was, and she said applesauce. Try these, you will love them!

2 cups (160 g) rolled oats
1 cup (125 g) all-purpose flour
½ cup (63 g) whole wheat flour
1 teaspoon baking soda
1 teaspoon ground cinnamon
½ teaspoon salt
**1 cup (245 g) *Pure Fuji Apple Purée*,
    page 125**
½ cup (170 g) honey
½ cup (100 g) pure cane sugar
1 egg, beaten
2 tablespoons (30 ml) coconut oil
**1 tablespoon (15 ml) vanilla
    extract**

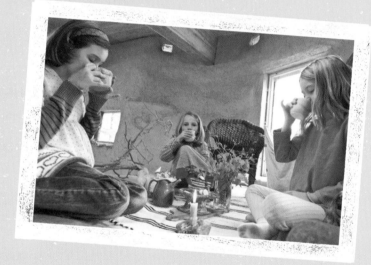

1. Preheat the oven to 350°F (180°C, or gas mark 4).
2. Combine oats, all-purpose flour, whole wheat flour, baking soda, cinnamon, and salt.
3. In a separate bowl, mix together remaining ingredients.
4. In a mixer, on low speed, add the flour mixture to the wet ingredients a little bit at a time until you have added it all and you have a doughlike batter.
5. On a parchment-lined baking sheet, spoon tablespoon scoops of cookie dough (about 1 tablespoon [16 g]) and flatten each one into a round.
6. Bake for 12 to 15 minutes until lightly browned, but still chewy.
7. Let cool on a wire rack and serve with your favorite milk.

Fruity Bread Pudding

15+ months

YIELD: 6 TO 10 SERVINGS

I love hitting the farmers' market. This is one of my very favorite outings. It's a place where every-thing seems right with the world. People are connecting, sharing, bartering, and living in harmony. The marketplace is especially delicious when it's bursting with these fall rustic flavors that bring forth traditional classics, such as bread pudding. I love food that has heart and soul, and bread pudding has that homespun energy about it that makes me feel like "love" is an actual ingredient needed to make this dish taste like my childhood.

6 thick slices brioche bread, cubed

2 tablespoons (28 g) unsalted butter, melted

4 eggs, beaten

2 cups (475 ml) milk

¾ cup (170 g) brown sugar

1 cup (250 g) *Spiced Apple, Pear, and Raisin Purée*, page 127

1. Preheat the oven to 350°F (180°C, or gas mark 4).
2. In an 8-inch (20 cm)-square baking dish, place cubed bread and drizzle with melted butter.
3. In a bowl, combine the eggs, milk, sugar, and *Spiced Apple, Pear, and Raisin Purée*.
4. Pour mixture evenly over bread, making sure the bread is soaking up the wet mixture (toss lightly if necessary).
5. Bake for 45 minutes, until browned. Serve warm.

RECIPE NOTE

This dish is great for breakfast or dessert. Top with yogurt, freshly whipped cream and fruit (as pictured), or whatever else you like.

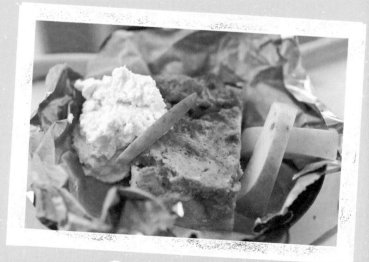

Crispy Baked Taquitos

15+ months

YIELD: 12 TAQUITOS, OR SERVINGS

....

These make a great midday snack and can be frozen if you want to make extra. My kids love easy-to-grab food and these are something they can snack on while playing, or you can bring some to the park for a nice, healthy, protein-packed snack on the go.

**2 cups (500 g) *Baby Refried Beans and Cheese*,
   page 128**
½ cup (60 g) grated cheddar cheese
½ cup (110 g) canned organic corn
12 corn tortillas
**1 tablespoon (15 ml) safflower oil
   (or your favorite cooking oil)**
Salsa or guacamole, for serving

1. Preheat the oven to 425°F (220°C, or gas mark 7).

2. In a large bowl, combine the *Baby Refried Beans and Cheese*, cheese, and corn. Set aside.

3. In a nonstick pan over medium heat, heat the corn tortillas until soft and pliable. Stack them on a plate and cover with a clean dish towel to keep warm.

4. Take a large spoonful of the bean mixture and place it down the middle of one of the tortillas. Roll up tightly, using a toothpick to keep in place if necessary. Place on a parchment-lined baking sheet.

5. Repeat with remaining tortillas and filling.

6. Brush taquitos with a little oil and bake for 10 to 15 minutes, or until crispy.

7. Serve warm with a side of salsa or guacamole.

Apple Pumpkin Butter

12+ months

YIELD: 3 TO 4 HALF-PINT (8-OUNCE, OR 235 ML) JARS

....

Pumpkin butter is good on so many things and it can be canned and used at a food swap or given out as a nice holiday gift. The flavors are so comforting—spread it on bread, waffles, dessert crêpes, or even vanilla bean ice cream topped with chopped walnuts.

**3 cups (750 g) *Ginger-Spiced Pumpkin Purée*,
   page 129**
**1 cup (250 g) applesauce or *Pure Fuji Apple
   Purée*, page 125**
½ cup (170 g) maple syrup
½ cup (170 g) raw agave nectar
½ lemon, squeezed
¼ teaspoon salt

1. In a large soup pot over medium heat, combine all the ingredients and bring to a boil, stirring frequently.

2. Reduce to low and let simmer about 20 to 25 minutes, until the butter thickens up.

3. Ladle into sterilized half-pint (8-ounce, or 235 ml)-glass jars. Let cool, then seal and date with the label.

4. Store in the refrigerator for up to a week.

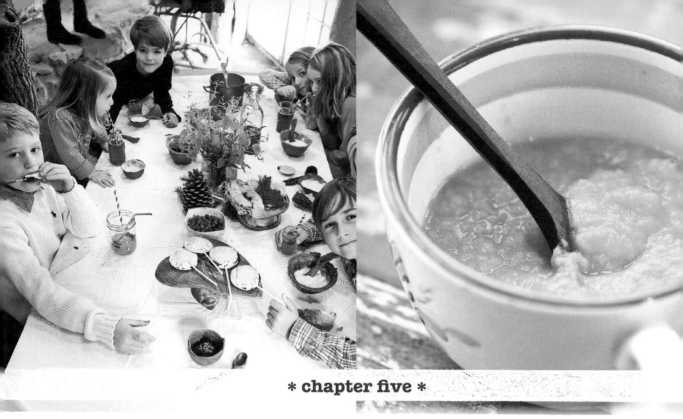

winter purées

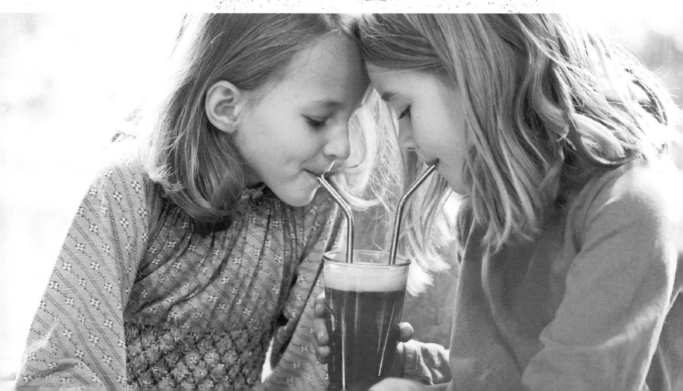

Welcome to winter, where the trees are bare, fires warm the home, and the cupboards are full of fall's excess bounty. This is the time when families come together for shared meals and celebrations and when grandmothers pass down cooking traditions long held sacred in the family. It is a time for both random and calculated generosity, where giving is the theme of the day.

What is amazing about having your own children is that you can start new traditions in these months—and throughout the year—based on your own food philosophy, and pass them down to your children as they grow throughout the years.

The Value of Sharing

Sharing food and friendship is what this time of year is all about. Fostering an environment of cozy dinner parties with family and friends sets up an environment of sharing and community for your baby and children. That translates into a happy home and healthy lifestyle. These early memories of having others over to share in meal times has a lasting impression on babies and inherently teaches them the value of food traditions and what it truly means to break bread together.

My husband and I like our children to bake breads and muffins and make comforting soups to share with those in need during the holiday season. Our kids take time and care in wrapping holiday breads and labeling huge mason jars filled with soup to give to our local homeless shelter. This act of giving teaches our children a sense of gratitude for what they have and a generosity of spirit that can only be fostered with actions and commitment to the greater good.

Allow Your Children to Cook with You!

Children love to help in the kitchen, and they can do a lot more than you might think. When my daughter turned seven, we had a party, and one of the dishes we served was a warm vegetable soup, as she is a fall child. Lotus cut every vegetable in that soup and was very proud to tell her friends all about it when they arrived for the party. We do homemade pizzas every week, and all the children, even my baby River, loves to roll out the dough and put the toppings on. This teaches them without "teaching," which is what I love, and it brings families together. Don't worry about the mess, and just let them play!

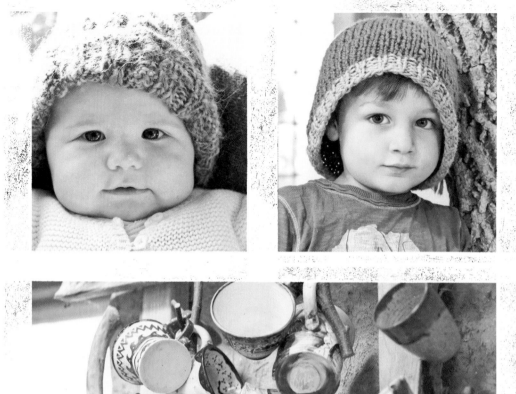

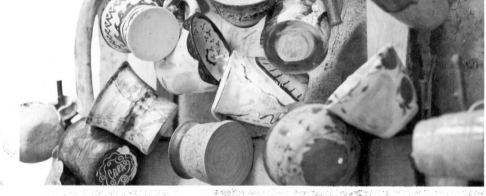

Winter Cleaning: Give Your Pantry a Makeover

I know most people advocate cleaning out in the spring, but I like to do this type of thing in the winter time. I find that I have more time indoors at home and want to get my kitchen restocked for the upcoming year. Cleaning and restocking the pantry is also helpful when preparing to make a bunch of purées because it ensures you have everything on hand, which makes the cooking process seamless and stress free.

If you are new to healthy eating and organic foods, you can also take this time to start replacing some of your old spices, cooking oils, and other products with refreshed, healthier versions.

The following is a short list of pantry suggestions I like to have on hand for healthy family cooking.

✳ COOKING OILS ✳

› Coconut oil
› Grapeseed oil
› Sunflower oil
› Olive oil

✳ SEASONINGS AND STOCKS ✳

› Whole garlic (keep in a cool, dark place)
› Yellow onions (keep in a cool, dark place)
› Sea salt
› Salts with minerals added in (colored salts)
› Pepper
› Bragg Liquid Aminos
› Low sodium soy sauce
› Tamari
› Thyme
› Oregano
› Chinese five-spice powder
› Cumin
› Cloves
› Turmeric
› Organic vegetable stock
› Organic chicken stock
› Organice beef stock

✳ BAKING PRODUCTS AND SWEETENERS ✳

› Various flours (all-purpose, whole wheat, etc.)
› Baking powder Make your own, if possible!)
› Vanilla extract
› Cocoa
› Coconut sugar
› Pure cane sugar
› Raw agave nectar
› Local honey

✳ GRAINS ✳

› Quinoa
› Millet
› Whole grain oats
› Brown rice
› Fresh granola

✳ DAIRY ✳

› Raw or organic milk
› Coconut milk
› Heavy cream
› Fresh butter
› Various types of cheeses
› Plain Greek yogurt

Babies Love Flavor!

Parents ask me all the time is, "Is it okay to give my baby spices, herbs, and flavors from my culture?" The answer is a simple and resounding "yes"! Just as adults prefer foods that have flavor, so do babies! This is how we help to shape their culinary palates. Babies eat what they are used to, and when you are pregnant, they get used to the flavors that you nourish yourself with. That is how early their relationship to food begins. Just be moderate in spicing up the food too much until they get used to eating. Add aromatics like onions and garlic to give bland purées a little kick. Adding flavor will help your baby start to develop a wide range of food preferences.

Roasted Vegetable Medley Purée

8+ months

YIELD: 5 CUPS (1.25 KG), OR 10 SERVINGS

2-IN-1 OPTION: **WINTER SQUASH SOUP**, PAGE 170

This is a fun dish because you can play with it depending on what you have in your garden or fridge at the time. I always say you can't go wrong as long as you have onions and garlic in your home. Remember that babies like flavor just as much as you do, so don't be shy about introducing your baby to the spices of life.

3 carrots, peeled and chopped

3 small yellow Finn potatoes, sliced into rounds

1 winter squash, halved and seeded

1 red onion, chopped

4 garlic gloves, minced

1. Preheat the oven to 350°F (180°C, or gas mark 4).
2. Place the carrots, potatoes, squash halves (face down), red onion, and garlic on a lined parchment baking sheet. Bake vegetables for 30 to 40 minutes, until soft.
3. Scoop the squash from the skin. Transfer squash and all other ingredients to a blender with ½ cup (120 ml) water and purée. Add more water as needed to obtain the desired consistency.

RECIPE NOTE

If you can't find yellow Finn potatoes, which have a very creamy, buttery flavor, substitute Yukon Gold.

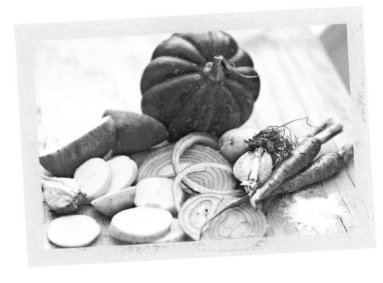

Beets and Berries Purée

9+ months

YIELD: 2 CUPS (500 G), OR 4 SERVINGS

2-IN-1 OPTION: **CHOCOLATE BEET CUPCAKES,** PAGE 171

....

Beets are so pretty and are full of vitamin B and magnesium. They are an acquired taste, and if you don't want to offer them alone, try this recipe with a little berry lovin' to sweeten the deal.

1 whole beet, peeled and cubed
1 cup (145 g) berries (raspberries, strawberries, or blackberries)

1. Steam the beet for 12 to 15 minutes, until soft.
2. Reserve the liquid from the steamer.
3. Purée the beet and raw berries in a food processor with ¼ cup (60 ml) of the reserved liquid. Add more liquid as needed to obtain the desired consistency.

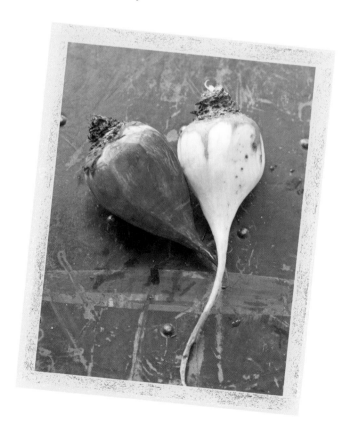

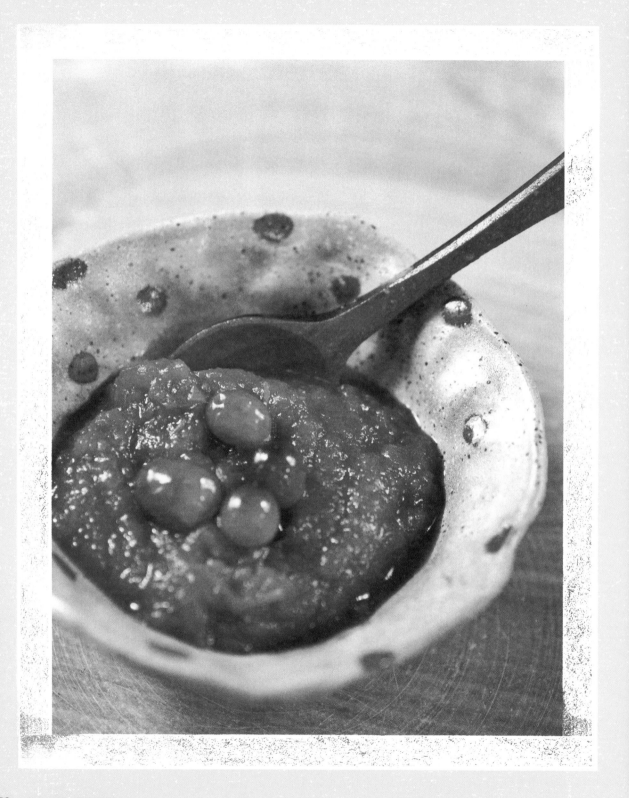

Cran-Apple Raisin Purée

7+ months

YIELD: 2½ CUPS (650 G), OR 4 BABY SERVINGS

2-IN-1 OPTION: **WHOLESOME BREAKFAST MUFFINS,** PAGE 172

....

This is a tart dish, but don't try to mask the flavor—it's okay to serve your baby foods with strong flavor profiles. This helps to balance their palates in a way that expands what their likes and dislikes may develop into.

1 cup (100 g) fresh cranberries
3 Fuji apples
½ cup (75 g) raisins
Juice of half a lemon (Meyer lemon, if possible)

1. Steam the cranberries and apples together for 8 to 10 minutes, or until soft.
2. Add the raisins and steam for 2 additional minutes. Reserve the liquid from the steamer.
3. Purée the cranberries, apple, and raisins in a food processor with ¼ cup of the reserved liquid and lemon juice. Add more liquid as needed to obtain the desired consistency.

RECIPE NOTE
....

Meyer lemons are a cross between a lemon and a mandarin orange and have a more nuanced tart flavor. They are rising in popularity, so keep any eye out for them and grab some when you find them!

Sweet Potato and Cashew Purée

9+ months

YIELD: 2½ CUPS (650 G), OR 4 TO 5 BABY SERVINGS

2-IN-1 OPTION: **SWEET POTATO MAPLE BUTTER** PAGE 173

Around the holidays, sweet potatoes are big in our home. We make sweet potatoes in all kinds of ways because everyone loves them so much. This recipes adds a touch of nutty flavor that gives this simple dish a twist that not only will your baby love, but will give her a little bit of the protein that she needs.

1 whole sweet potato, peeled and cubed

½ cup (75 g) unsalted cashews, ground to a powder in your coffee grinder

1. Steam the sweet potatoes for 12 to 15 minutes, or until soft. Reserve the liquid from the steamer.
2. Purée the sweet potatoes in a food processor with ¼ cup (60 ml) of the reserved liquid and cashew powder. Add more liquid as needed to obtain the desired consistency.

What about Juice?

There is no need to start your baby on juice, and especially not before she turns one. Manufacturers add so much sugar to their juices that they are hardly worth buying. Even the ones that say "no sugar added" have been highly processed and are not great for kids.

If you want to offer your children an alternative to water, which of course is the best drink option, try herbal teas. Herbal teas are not really teas at all, because they contain no caffeine. They are really the essence of wildflowers. Sweeten the drinks with a little local honey, and you have a nice refreshing drink. Try mint lemon, rooibos chamomile, or a refreshing peach tea, and you also boost your children's immunity and get them used to a less sugary tasting drinks.

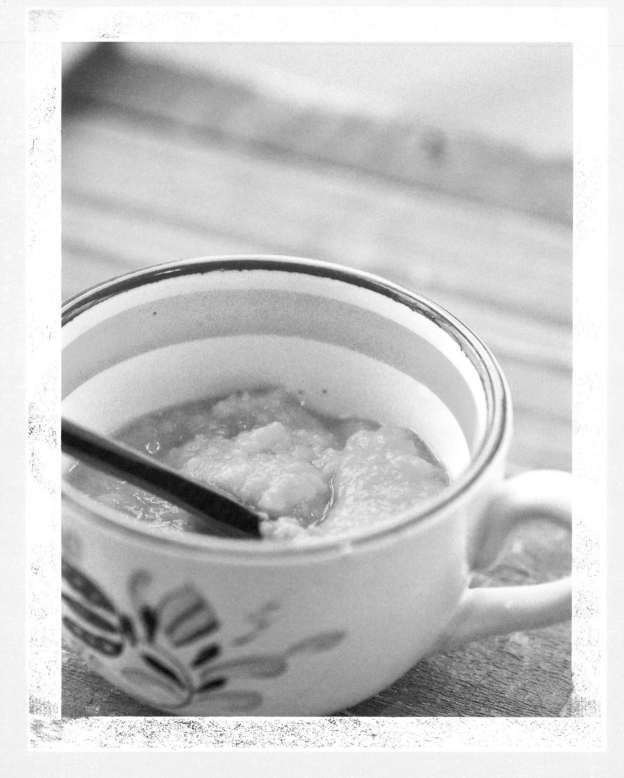

Apple, Sweet Potato, and Tomato Chutney Textured Meal

12+ months (due to the honey in this recipe)

YIELD: ABOUT 4 CUPS (1 KG), OR 6 SERVINGS

2-IN-1 OPTION: **INDIAN-SPICED COUSCOUS,** PAGE 174

My kids love Indian food, as they have eaten it since they were babies. The flavors of sweet and savory play well with babies, and it's fun to introduce them to unique flavor profiles that will help build an adventurous palate. This is a delicious baby food recipe that you can also serve with crackers and olives at parties.

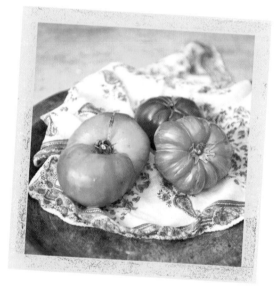

6 apples, peeled and cut

6 tomatoes, peeled and chopped

½ small sweet potato, peeled and chopped

2 large yellow onions, chopped

2 garlic cloves, minced

1 cup (178 g) pitted dates, chopped

2 teaspoons (5 g) ground cardamom

2 teaspoons (4 g) turmeric

2 teaspoons (5 g) ground cumin

2 cups (680 g) honey

2 cups (400 g) natural cane sugar, such as Sucanat

1 tablespoon (7 g) wheat germ

1 teaspoon sea salt

½ teaspoon pepper

2 cups (475 ml) distilled vinegar

1. In a large soup pot, combine all the ingredients. Bring to a boil, reduce heat, and simmer, stirring frequently, for 45 to 50 minutes until the mixture becomes pulpy and thick.

RECIPE NOTE

Spoon the chutney into clear glass jars for storage and seal with an airtight lid. This recipe will last for up to four weeks refrigerated.

winter purées

Cheesy Cauliflower Purée

12+ months

YIELD: 3 CUPS (750 G), OR 5 BABY SERVINGS

2-IN-1 OPTION: **CHEESY CAULIFLOWER-STUFFED POTATOES,** PAGE 174

....

Cauliflower is a nice purée for baby, and its mild flavor lends itself well to a cheesy counterpart. It is also high in vitamin C and dietary fiber, so offering this to your baby with make you feel good knowing you and Mother Nature are working hand in hand to provide your baby the best nutrition possible.

2 cups (200 g) cauliflower florets, chopped
½ cup (120 ml) heavy cream
½ cup (60 g) shredded Gruyére cheese
½ cup (60 g) shredded sharp Cheddar cheese
¼ teaspoon nutmeg

1. Steam the cauliflower for 10 to 12 minutes, until soft.

2. Reserve the liquid from the steamer.

3. In a small pot on medium heat, combine the cream, cheeses, and nutmeg and cook until melted together.

4. Purée the cauliflower with the cheese mixture and ¼ cup (60 ml) of the reserved liquid. Add more liquid as needed to obtain the desired consistency.

winter purées

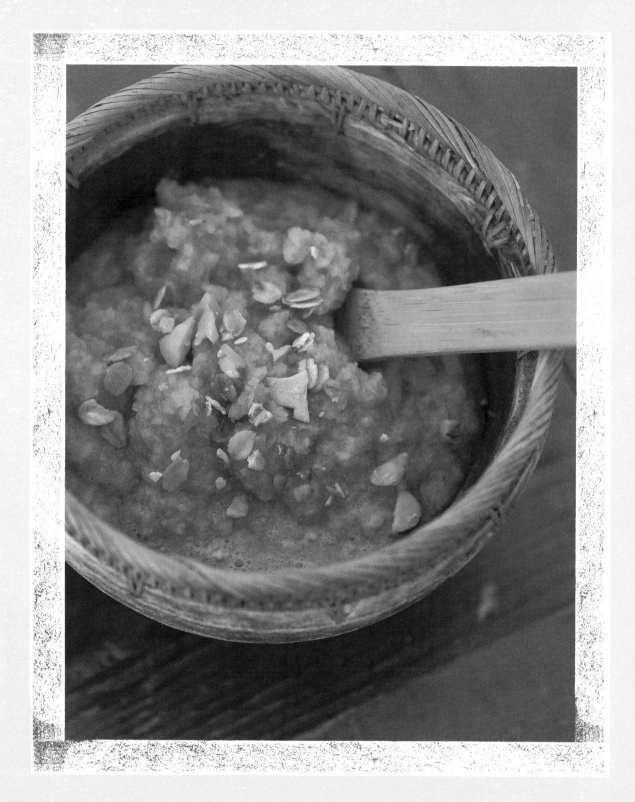

Multigrain Fruit and Nut Textured Meal

12+ months

YIELD: 10 CUPS (2.5 KG), OR 20 BABY SERVINGS

2-IN-1 OPTION: **APPLE PECAN PROTEIN BISCUITS,** PAGE 175

This is a warm, slow-cooker breakfast that babies and older kids love. This does not have to be a meal just for your littlest love in the house. Serve it up to everyone in your home, and send them off for the day with warm and satisfied bellies.

1 pear, peeled and diced small
3 Fuji apples, peeled and diced small
1 cup (80 g) steel-cut oats, uncooked
1 cup (185 g) millet, uncooked
1 cup (175 g) quinoa, uncooked
1 teaspoon wheat germ
1 teaspoon ground flaxseed
2½ cups (570 ml) soymilk
5 cups (1.25 L) water
1 cup (145 g) raisins
½ cup (110 g) chopped pecans

1. Place all of the ingredients in a slow cooker and cook overnight on low for up to 8 hours.
2. Serve warm in the morning for breakfast.

Broccoli, Leek, and Basil Purée

9+ months

YIELD: 2½ (650 G) CUPS, OR 5 BABY SERVINGS

2-IN-1 OPTION: **FLANK STEAK TACOS WITH AIOLI,** PAGE 176

....

I love adding fresh aromatics to baby food. They freshen up meals and offer fun and unique flavor twists that naturally expand a baby's palate. Basil is a wonderful herb that is traditionally used in many Italian dishes, but it can be easily paired with a wide variety of dishes. It has anti-bacterial properties and is high in iron.

1 cup (70 g) broccoli, chopped small

1 small leek, chopped small

1 cup (40 g) fresh chopped basil

1. Steam broccoli and leek for 7 to 10 minutes, until soft. Reserve the water from the steamer.

2. Purée the broccoli, leek, and basil in a blender or food processor. Add 1 teaspoon (5 ml) of reserved water at a time, if necessary, until desired consistency is achieved.

Quick and Healthy Snack Ideas for Kids

> Whole wheat crackers with honey butter
> Apple slices with almond butter
> Yogurt with a purée mixed in and topped with granola
> Broccoli with freshly grated and melted cheese sauce
> Whole grain chips and salsa
> Kale popcorn or crispy kale chips
> Veggie ice pops (check out my book, *Ice Pop Joy*, for more great ice pop ideas)
> Cheese, freshly cut salami, and wholegrain crackers with sunflower honey
> Various olives (no pits)

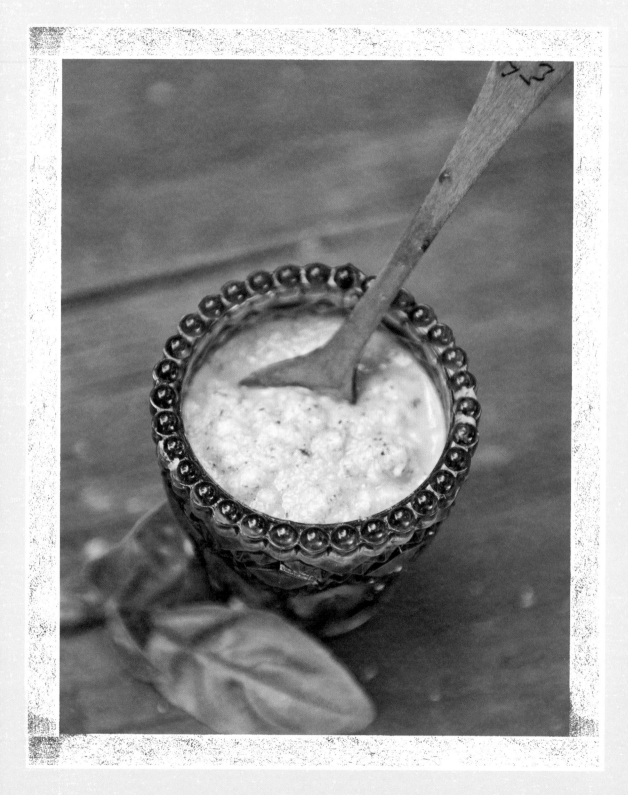

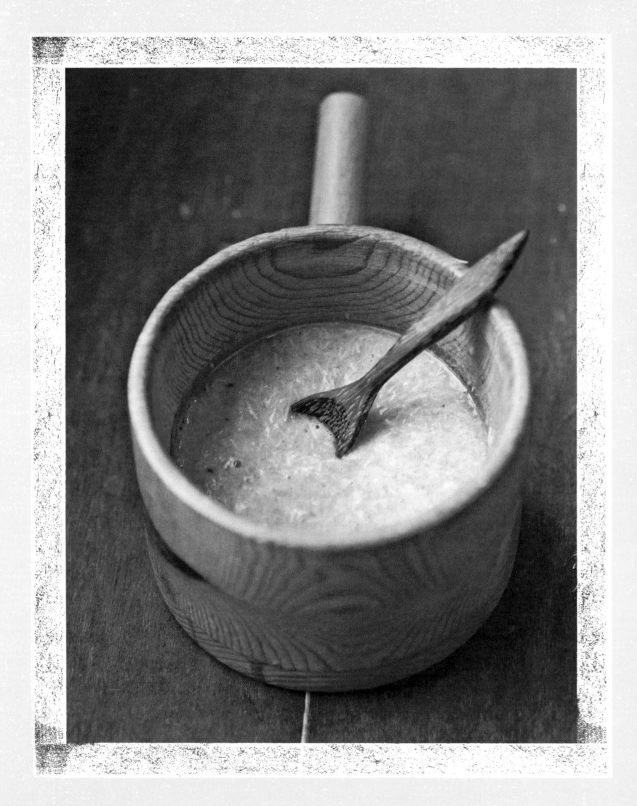

Chicken and Veggie Textured Meal

10+ months

YIELD: 5 CUPS (1.25 KG), OR 10 BABY SERVINGS

2-IN-1 OPTION: **CHICKEN AND ECHINACEA SOUP,** PAGE 177

....

As much fun as the winter season brings, there is also the inevitable cold and flu that little ones seem to drag home from all over town. Warm chicken soup is what most mom-doctors order up when this season hits home. When you add in your mommy touch, you boost your children's immunity a ton! I can't prove that, but I know it's true. Love goes a long way.

6 cups (1.5 L) water
1 small chicken (preferably organic)
1 carrot, chopped
1 yellow onion, chopped
1 celery stalk, chopped
2 garlic gloves, minced
2 sprigs fresh thyme
1 large helping of Mom's love

1. In a large soup pot, boil water. Add the whole chicken, carrot, yellow onion, celery, garlic, and thyme.

2. Reduce to a simmer and let cook for 35 to 45 minutes, until the chicken is cooked and the meat is falling off of the bone.

3. Let this mixture cool. Strain half of the broth into another bowl and refrigerate for future use.

4. Take the whole chicken out of the pot and pull all of the meat off. Place the meat back into the pot.

5. Transfer the contents of the pot to the blender (working in batches if you need to) and blend to a consistency your baby can handle, adding additional broth as necessary.

6. Don't forget to add the love! (That is the secret ingredient.)

winter purées

Pure Kale Purée

7+ months

YIELD: 3 CUPS (750 G), OR 5 BABY SERVINGS

2-IN-1 OPTION: **COMFORTING POTATO AND KALE GRATIN,** PAGE 178

. . . .

Kale is a super green that kids need. I love serving "crispy kale" to my children for an afternoon snack. All you do is preheat the oven to 350°F (180°C, or gas mark 4), season fresh kale with salt and pepper, and bake for 8 to 10 minutes until crispy. Sprinkle with parmesan cheese before you bake it, and your kids will go crazy for it!

3 cups (200 g) fresh kale, chopped

1. Steam the kale for 10 minutes, or until soft. Reserve the liquid from the steamer.
2. Purée the kale in a blender or food processor with 2 tablespoons (28 ml) of the reserved liquid. Add more liquid as needed to obtain the desired consistency.

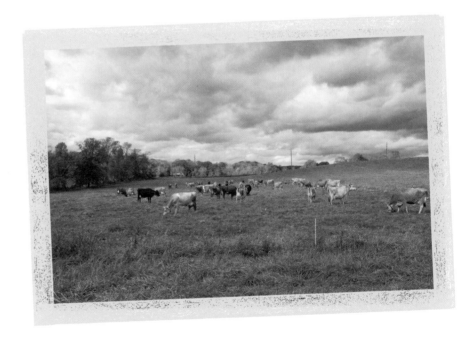

Pure Plum Purée

6+ months

YIELD: 3 CUPS (750 G), OR 5 BABY SERVINGS

2-IN-1 OPTION: **ORANGE PLUM ITALIAN ICE,** PAGE 178

....

Plums are sweet and full of fiber and vitamin C. This is a baby classic, and I do not think I have ever met a baby who did not go crazy for just plain old plums. Try using this purée to make fruit leather: simply place a thin layer of the purée on a baking sheet and let it cook overnight on the lowest temperature your oven will go. If it won't set, just as a lovely sauce for a winter pancake morning!

5 fresh plums, chopped, skins on

1. Steam the plums for 5 to 7 minutes, or until soft. Reserve the liquid from the steamer.
2. Purée the plums with 2 tablespoons (28 ml) of the reserved liquid. Add more liquid as needed to obtain the desired consistency.

Bolognese Textured Meal

11+ months

YIELD: 6 CUPS (1.5 KG), OR 12 BABY SERVINGS

2-IN-1 OPTION: **LASAGNA BOLOGNESE,** PAGE 179

Bolognese is a classic Italian meal that almost everyone loves. There is something about it that is warm and comforting, and in those winter months of spending more time inside, it's a welcome feast. When it's cooking, it smells delicious, and I find that it literally lures all the folks in the home into the kitchen. Every time I make this, my baby goes crazy, and my 4-year-old son Bodhi always says, "What is that delicious smell, Mama?" Of course, you can easily add this sauce to a batch of spaghetti for a meal the whole family will love.

1 tablespoon (15 ml) coconut oil
1 pound (450 g) lean ground beef
1 yellow onion, finely chopped
3 garlic cloves, minced
1 cup (40 g) finely chopped fresh basil
¼ cup (15 g) finely chopped fresh parsley
2 large tomatoes, cut in chunks
1 can (8 ounces or 226 g) tomato sauce
½ teaspoon garlic powder
½ teaspoon sea salt
½ teaspoon pepper
1 teaspoon wheat germ

1. In a large skillet, heat coconut oil over medium heat. Add beef and partially brown.
2. Add onion and garlic cloves and cook until onions are translucent.
3. Add basil, parsley, tomatoes, tomato sauce, seasonings, and wheat germ.
4. Bring to a boil and simmer 20 to 25 minutes.
5. Mash with a wooden spoon if necessary, to reach desired consistency for baby. Serve warm.

winter purées

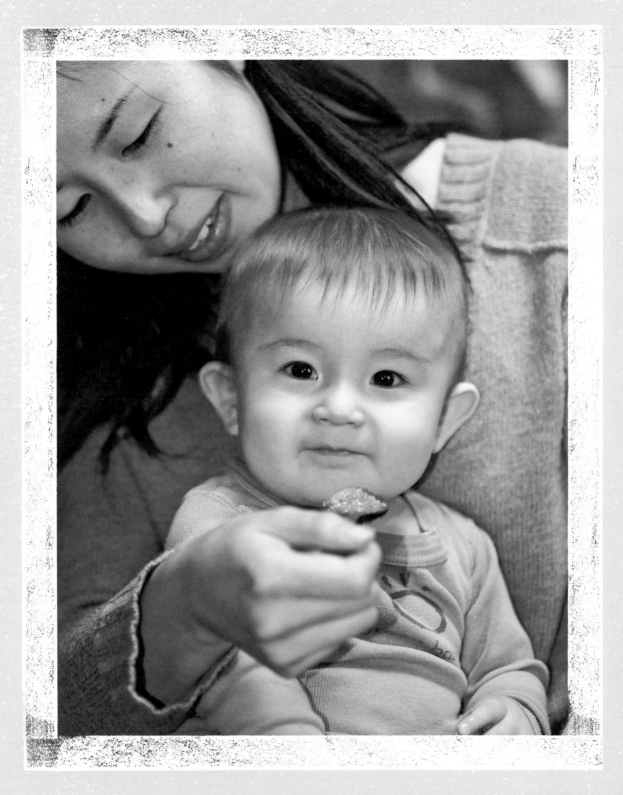

Hummus Purée

9+ months

YIELD: 2 CUPS, OR 8 BABY OR KID SERVINGS

2-IN-1 OPTION: **MOZZARELLA, TOMATO, AND BASIL PANINI,** PAGE 180

Hummus is a tasty way to get Baby some needed protein. This recipe has a great flavor profile for your baby to get accustomed to because it makes a protein-packed lunch for school days when he is older. Hummus lends itself well to added flavors, such as nuts, olives, or other vegetables. You can also serve it to your older kids topped with roasted pine nuts and warm pita bread.

1 can (14 ounces or 396 g) garbanzo beans, drained
3 garlic gloves, minced
1 tablespoon (15 ml) olive oil
3 tablespoons (45 ml) lemon juice

1. Purée all ingredients in blend or food processor until smooth.

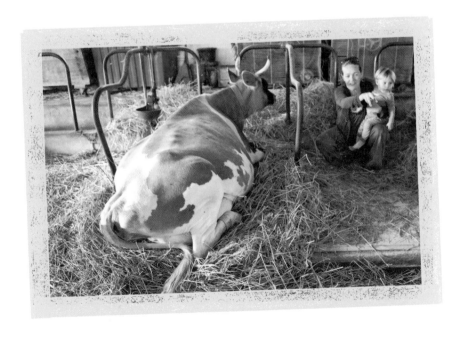

Bright Corn Purée

9+ months

YIELD: 2 TO 3 CUPS (500 TO 750 G), OR 4 TO 6 BABY SERVINGS

2-IN-1 OPTION: **SAUSAGE AND CORN BREAKFAST BAKE**, PAGE 180

Fresh corn is sweet and savory, and babies love it. I know corn is at its freshest in the summer in most areas, but if you're lucky enough to have access to it throughout the year, it's so worth it. Frozen corn is also a perfectly acceptable substitute. Frozen vegetables have been picked at the peak of their ripeness and immediately flash frozen, so all of their nutrients remain intact.

4 ears of fresh corn, shucked*
½ cup (120 ml) vegetable broth

1. In a large pot, boil the corn on the cob for 9 minutes.
2. Allow corn to cool. Cut all of the corn off the ears and so you are left with only the kernels.
3. Combine the kernels with vegetable broth and purée in a blender or food processor to desired consistency.

RECIPE NOTES

› *If using frozen, simple substitute one 10-ounce package (285 g) whole-kernel corn for the fresh. No need to defrost.
› If you have any leftover corn kernels, throw some in a simple green salad the next day for an added flavor boost and a fun twist.

Sweet Potato, Prosciutto, and Cheese Purée

12+ months

YIELD: 4 TO 5 CUPS (1 TO 1.25 KG), OR 8 BABY SERVINGS

2-IN-1 OPTION: **BREAKFAST WAFFLES FOR DINNER,** PAGE 181

Caregivers, you will love this one yourself, so be sure to make extra to share with baby. These flavors meld so well together and bring this sweet and savory combination to a new level for baby food. Older children love this too, so make sure to share!

2 sweet potatoes, halved
4 strips of prosciutto
½ cup (60 g) grated gruyere cheese

1. Preheat your oven to 400°F (200°C, or gas mark 6).
2. Bake the sweet potatoes about 40 minutes, until soft.
3. Place the strips of prosciutto on the baking sheet, next to the sweet potatoes, for the last 5 minutes of cooking and cook until crisp.
4. Once cool enough to handle, scoop out the insides of the sweet potato into the blender bowl.
5. Add prosciutto, cheese, and ¼ cup (60 ml) of water, and purée until the desired consistency is achieved.

winter purées

Cranberry, Pomegranate, and Greek Yogurt Purée

9+ months

YIELD: 3 CUPS (750 G), OR 6 TO 8 BABY SERVINGS

2-IN-1 OPTION: **SWEET AND CREAMY WINTER ICE POPS,** PAGE 181

This little combination is high in antioxidants and protein and has the needed healthy probiotics for your baby's brain to develop. All that in just one little purée—and it tastes so good! When your baby gets a little older, consider adding some chopped nuts to this yogurt, and you will really have a powerhouse of nutrition on your hands.

1 cup (100 g) fresh or frozen cranberries
1 whole fresh pomegranate, seeded
1½ cups of plain (345 g) Greek yogurt

1. Steam the cranberries for about 7 to 10 minutes, or until soft. Reserve the liquid from the steamer.
2. Purée the cranberries with the pomegranate seeds and 2 tablespoons (28 ml) of the reserved liquid.
3. Add the Greek yogurt and blend until desired consistency is achieved.

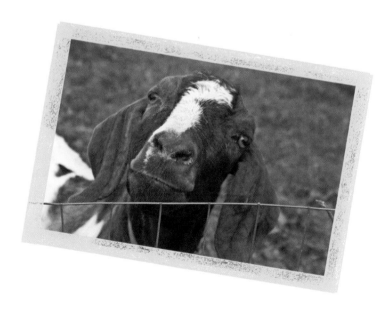

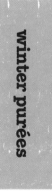
winter purées

Winter Squash Soup

15+ months

YIELD: 8 CUPS (2 KG), OR 10 SERVINGS

When the cold blows into my area in Chester Springs, Pennsylvania, we have very crisp mornings and afternoons after school. This is a time of year when soup is the perfect food. It's nourishing, warm, filling, and super tasty. Squash are always fun for kids to grow in the garden too, because they get to watch them get huge, and soups are a great way to put that bounty to use and give your kids a nice shot of vitamin A and C.

1 tablespoon (15 ml) extra-virgin olive oil

1 yellow onion, chopped

3 cloves garlic, chopped

4 cups (980 g) *Roasted Vegetable Medley Purée*, page 148

1 can (32 ounces or 1 L) chicken broth

½ cup (120 ml) coconut milk

¼ teaspoon freshly grated nutmeg

¼ teaspoon sea salt

¼ teaspoon pepper

Roasted pine nuts, for topping

2 tablespoons (30 g) ricotta cheese, for topping

Cinnamon, for sprinkling

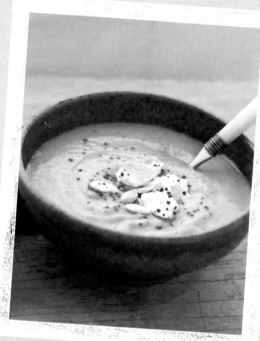

1. In a soup pot over medium heat, heat oil. Add onion and garlic and sauté for 8 to 10 minutes.

2. Add the *Roasted Vegetable Medley Purée* and stir to combine.

3. Add chicken broth and coconut milk. Season with nutmeg, salt, and pepper. Bring to a boil.

4. Reduce heat and simmer for 15 to 20 minutes until the flavors meld well together.

5. While soup is simmering, toast a handful of pine nuts in a sauté pan on low heat. Constantly shake the pine nuts around in the pan until lightly browned, being careful not to burn. Set aside.

6. Using a blender, purée your soup to a smooth and silky texture.

7. Top with pine nuts, a scoop of ricotta, and a slight sprinkle of cinnamon.

Chocolate Beet Cupcakes

18+ months

YIELD: 12 TO 15 CUPCAKES, OR SERVINGS

We love cupcakes in our house, and this recipe makes them extra nutritious and tasty with the added *Beets and Berries Purée*. These cupcakes are fun for birthday parties or just a nice after school project for older kids. My daughter Lotus says that beets look like roses, so she is happy to make anything with them!

1 cup (125 g) all-purpose flour
¾ teaspoon baking soda
¼ teaspoon baking powder
¼ teaspoon sea salt
3 ounces (85 g) dark organic chocolate, chopped
½ cup (112 g) unsalted butter
1 cup (200 g) pure cane sugar
1 egg, beaten
1 cup (245 g) *Beets and Berries Purée*, page 149

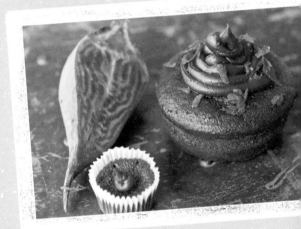

1. Preheat oven to 350°F (180° C, or gas mark 4).
2. In a large mixing bowl, combine the flour, baking soda, baking powder, and salt.
3. Place the chopped chocolate and butter in a stainless steel bowl and place bowl over a pot of boiling water, making sure the bowl doesn't touch the water. Let the butter and chocolate melt together, then remove from heat.
4. Add the sugar to the chocolate mixture and mix well.
5. Fold in egg and *Beets and Berries Purée*.
6. Fold in the flour mixture.
7. Line a cupcake pan with liners and fill each one about three-quarters of the way full.
8. Bake for 20 to 25 minutes until toothpick inserted in the center comes out clean.
9. Let cool on a wire rack and serve warm.

RECIPE NOTES

› Feel free to frost with your favorite icing or whipped cream—just be sure to let the cupcakes cool for at least 20 minutes before doing so.

› Use this recipe to make any size cakes you like. Grease and flour your pans first to prevent sticking, and keep an eye on your baking time, as it will vary depending on what size pan you're using. The toothpick test will be a reliable indicator of doneness.

Wholesome Breakfast Muffins

13+ months

YIELD: 6 TO 8 BAKERY SIZE MUFFINS, OR SERVINGS

....

Breakfast muffins are a great way to start the day. You can make them the night before for a quick bite before school. As you can see from the picture, our little buddy Ryan loved these muffins and kept coming back for more!

2 cups (250 g) whole wheat pastry flour
1 teaspoon baking soda
2 teaspoons (5 g) cinnamon
1 teaspoon fresh nutmeg
½ teaspoon sea salt
½ cup (112 g) unsalted butter, softened
1 cup (200 g) pure cane sugar
3 eggs
1½ cups (375 g) Cran-Apple Raisin Purée, page 151
½ cup (60 g) chopped walnuts, plus a few more for topping

1. Preheat the oven to 350°F (180°C, or gas mark 4).
2. Combine all dry ingredients.
3. In a separate bowl, using either a handheld or stand mixer on medium speed, beat butter with the sugar.
4. Beat in the eggs, one at a time.
5. Add the *Cran-Apple Raisin Purée* and chopped walnuts.
6. On low speed, add the flour mixture a little bit at a time, until you have added it all and you have a cake-like batter. Make sure no streaks of flour remain, but be careful not to overmix.
7. Line a jumbo muffin pan with cupcake liners and distribute batter equally, filling each about three-quarters full. Top with the reserved walnuts, if desired.
8. Bake 18 to 20 minutes, or until a toothpick inserted in the center comes out clean.
9. Cool slightly and serve warm.

RECIPE NOTE
....

Feel free to use a regular-sized muffin tin and liners if that's what you have. You'll get a few more muffins than the yield here—just be sure to keep an eye on the baking time, as they may require a few minutes less in the oven.

Sweet Potato Maple Butter

13+ months

YIELD: 2 CUPS (450 G)

....

We have an amazing dairy farm in our neighborhood called Seven Stars Farm. We have gotten to know the folks over there and even my little 4-year-old Bodhi goes over to pet the baby cows. He has a favorite named Pearl, born with a heart-shaped pattern on her head. Making homemade butter is the easiest thing in the world, but you have to start with fresh cream. The cream we get at Seven Stars is so amazing it's hard to put into words. When the cows are treated with love and kindness and are not stressed out, they produce happier, creamier products.

2 cups (475 ml) heavy cream
¼ cup (85 g) pure maple syrup
½ cup (125 g) *Sweet Potato and Cashew Purée*, page 152
½ teaspoon sea salt
Bread, for serving

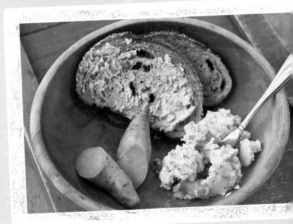

1. In a large mixer, whip the cream, maple syrup, and salt on high for 10 minutes.

2. Reduce to medium speed and continue whipping, past the whipped cream stage, until it turns into a ball of butter and the buttermilk separates from it.

3. Pour off the butter milk and set aside.

4. Add the *Sweet Potato and Cashew Purée* to the butter and whip on medium speed until nicely blended.

5. Transfer the ball of butter from the mixer to a cheesecloth or light linen cloth.

6. Wrap the cloth around the butter and squeeze it to remove excess liquid. Shape to desired shape or leave in a rustic ball.

7. Serve on warm bread and refrigerate remainder. Keep the buttermilk in a glass mason jar in the fridge for future recipes (or drink as is—it's full of healthy enzymes!).

RECIPE NOTES

....

> Adapt this recipe to make roasted garlic butter or honey butter! The only thing that's essential is the heavy cream, so feel free to swap in or out whatever ingredients you like.

> Include your kids in the butter making process—they will love to see it go from cream, to whipped cream, to butter, to buttermilk. Plus they can taste at every stage!

Indian-Spiced Couscous

15+ months

YIELD: 4 CUPS, OR 4 ADULT SERVINGS, OR 4 TO 6 KID SERVINGS

....

Couscous is the easiest thing to make, and when you add the delicious chutney, you have a fun meal for the whole family. Serve this with some warm garlic naan bread, which you can now buy at the grocery store, and you have one terrific dish.

2½ cups (600 ml) water

2 cups (475 ml) vegetable broth

1 tablespoon (14 g) unsalted butter

3 cups (525 g) couscous, uncooked

2 cups *Apple, Sweet Potato, and Tomato Chutney Textured Meal*, page 154

Garlic naan, for serving

1. In a pot with a lid, bring the water, vegetable broth, and butter to a boil.

2. Add the couscous and stir. Remove the pot from the heat. Let the couscous sit, covered, for about 5 minutes until it absorbs the water mixture. Fluff with a fork. It should be soft and fluffy.

3. Mix the couscous with the *Apple, Sweet Potato, and Tomato Chutney Textured Meal.*

4. Serve with warm garlic naan.

Cheesy Cauliflower-Stuffed Potatoes

15+ months

YIELD: 4 ADULT SERVINGS OR 8 KID SERVINGS

....

Everyone loves stuffed potatoes. They are hearty and homey, and they just plain taste good. I like to make these for my family on "App Night," when we just have appetizers for dinner—kind of like tapas for kids. My friend Rachel came up with the concept, and we love it!

4 Russet potatoes

1 cup (245 g) *Cheesy Cauliflower Purée*, page 155

½ cup (50 g) grated parmesan cheese

¼ cup (60 g) sour cream

¼ cup (15 g) chopped chives

1 cup (80 g) baked, chopped prosciutto (like bacon bits)

Sea salt and pepper to taste

1. Preheat oven to 375°F (190°C, or gas mark 5). Bake potatoes for 50 to 60 minutes until soft.

2. Cut the potatoes in half (careful, they're hot!) and scoop out the insides, leaving just a little attached to the skin, so that you can easily put the stuffed potato mixture back into its shell.

3. Place the potato shells in a ceramic dish and bake for 15 minutes to crisp up while you prepare the potato filling.

4. In a bowl, combine the potato mash, *Cheesy Cauliflower Purée*, Parmesan cheese, sour cream, and chives. Season with salt and pepper.

5. Scoop the mixture into the individual shells and top with the prosciutto. Reheat in the oven for a few minutes if necessary and serve hot.

Apple Pecan Protein Biscuits

18+ months

YIELD: 25 BISCUITS, OR SERVINGS

....

These protein-packed biscuit cookies are tasty and healthy. They are my little River's favorites. We all try hard to get our children to eat well, and when they do, it brings us as parents such joy. Encourage your kiddos to eat these, and everyone will feel good as a result.

1 cup (125 g) all-purpose flour
½ cup (68 g) whole wheat flour
1 teaspoon baking soda
1 teaspoon ground cinnamon
½ teaspoon salt
2 cups (500 g) *Multigrain Fruit and Nut Textured Meal*, page 157
1 cup (340 g) honey
1 egg, beaten
2 tablespoons (30 ml) coconut oil
1 tablespoon (15 ml) vanilla extract
Chopped pecans, for topping (optional)

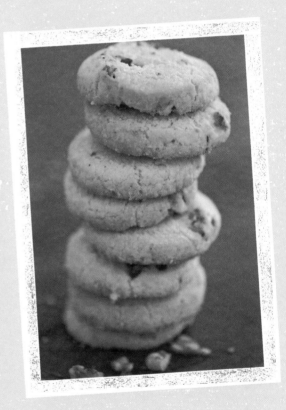

1. Preheat the oven to 350°F (180°C, or gas mark 4).
2. Combine dry ingredients.
3. In a blender, puree the *Multigrain Fruit and Nut Textured Meal* to a smooth texture.
4. In a separate bowl, combine the purée, honey, egg, coconut oil, and vanilla extract.
5. Add the flour mixture in a little bit at a time, until you have added it all and you have a dough-like batter.
6. On a parchment-lined baking pan, spoon 1 tablespoon (15 g) scoops of dough and flatten each one into a round. If you would like them in perfect biscuit circles, use a small round cookie cutter to shape.
7. Top each biscuit with chopped pecans, if desired.
8. Bake for 12 to 15 minutes until lightly browned.
9. Let cool on a wire rack before serving.

Flank Steak Tacos with Aioli

17+ months

YIELD: 6 SERVINGS

....

Taco night is big time fun in my house, and it is a great meal to invite friends over to share. Hosting a taco bar, where folks can make they own creations, is always fun and the twist of the aioli makes these tacos amazing!

FOR AIOLI:

6 garlic cloves

½ teaspoon sea salt

6 egg yolks

1 teaspoon Dijon mustard

¼ cup (60 g) *Broccoli, Leek, and Basil Purée*, page 158

1½ cups (355 ml) olive oil

FOR TACOS:

2 tablespoons (30 ml) coconut oil, divided

1 large red onion, sliced

2 pounds (900 g) flank steak

¼ teaspoon sea salt

¼ teaspoon pepper

12 to 14 corn tortillas, warmed

1 cup (150 g) halved grape tomatoes

1 cup (150 g) crumbled feta cheese

TO MAKE AIOLI:

1. In a blender, combine garlic cloves, sea salt, egg yolks, mustard, and *Broccoli, Leek, and Basil Purée*. Purée while very slowly streaming in the olive oil. Set aside until tacos are ready.

TO MAKE TACOS:

1. Preheat the oven to 425°F (220°C, or gas mark 7).

2. In a medium sauté pan, heat 1 tablespoon (15 ml) coconut oil and sauté red onion until caramelized, 7 to 10 minutes. Set aside.

3. Season the flank steak with salt and pepper on both sides.

4. Heat remaining tablespoon (15 ml) coconut oil in a cast iron sauté pan on medium heat. Sear the steak for 7 minutes on both sides.

5. Immediately place the cast iron pan in the oven for an additional 5 minutes.

6. Remove from oven and let the flank steak rest for a few minutes before cutting. Once rested, slice across the grain on the diagonal, about ¼-inch (6 mm)-thick.

7. Assemble tacos by dividing steak among warm tortillas and topping with sautéed red onions, grape tomatoes, and feta cheese.

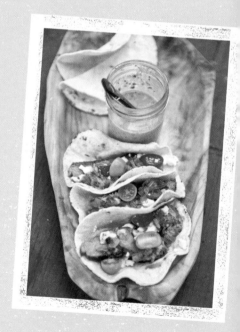

Chicken and Echinacea Soup

15+ months

YIELD: 8 CUPS, OR 10 SERVINGS

This soup takes the purée we started for baby and kicks it up a notch. It includes a shot of echinacea, a liquid herbal extract, to give everyone an immunity boost, which is so important during the winter months. Make this soup when your family needs a little special touch from Mama because they are feeling under the weather.

8 to 10 cups (2 to 2.5 L) water

1 small chicken

2 carrots, chopped

1 large yellow onion, chopped

2 celery stalks, chopped

2 garlic gloves, minced

2 sprigs fresh thyme

1 teaspoon sea salt

1 teaspoon pepper

1 tablespoon (15 ml) low sodium soy sauce

2 chicken bouillon cubes

1 teaspoon echinacea (I like Children's Echinacea by Herb Pharm)

2 cups (500 g) *Chicken and Veggie Textured Meal*, page 161

1. In a large soup pot, boil water. Add in the whole chicken, carrots, yellow onion, celery, garlic, thyme, salt, pepper, soy sauce, and chicken bouillon cubes.

2. Reduce heat to a simmer and let cook for 35 to 45 minutes, until the chicken is cooked and the meat is falling off of the bone.

3. Take the whole chicken out of the pot and tear all of the meat off. Place the meat back into the pot. Add in the echinacea and *Chicken and Veggie Textured Meal*.

4. Let the soup simmer on low to medium heat until ready to serve.

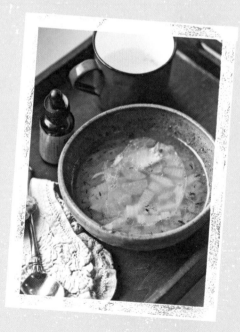

Comforting Potato and Kale Gratin

15+ months

YIELD: 4 ADULT SERVINGS OR 6 KID SERVINGS

....

This meal is so comforting because it reminds me of my childhood. This is still my go-to dish when I want to pay homage to my mama in my own cooking.

2 tablespoons (28 g) unsalted butter
5 red potatoes, sliced thin with a mandolin slicer
2 garlic cloves, minced
1 teaspoon sea salt
1 teaspoon pepper
1 teaspoon paprika
1 cup (120 g) shredded Cheddar cheese
1 cup (100 g) grated Parmesan cheese
1 cup (120 g) shredded sharp white Cheddar cheese
1 cup (245 g) *Pure Kale Purée* (page 162)
1 cup (235 ml) heavy cream
1 cup (235 ml) milk

1. Preheat oven to 375°F (190°C, or gas mark 5). Coat a 9 x 13-inch (22.8 x 33 cm) baking dish with the butter.

2. Arrange one-third of the sliced potatoes in a layer on the bottom of the dish. Sprinkle the potatoes with one-third of the garlic, salt, pepper, paprika, cheeses, and one-third of the *Pure Kale Purée*.

3. Repeat the layering process two additional times, ending with the purée.

4. Combine the cream and milk and slowly pour it over the potato mixture, distributing evenly.

5. Cover the dish with aluminum foil and bake for 25 to 30 minutes. Remove foil and bake an additional 7 minutes.

6. Let rest 15 to 20 minutes before cutting.

Orange Plum Italian Ice

14+ months

YIELD: 4 TO 5 SERVINGS

....

Yum is really all I can say here. Italian ice goes a long way in my family, as everyone loves it, especially when they are not feeling well. My son Zoe makes great Italian ices, and this one is the perfect combination of sweet and tart.

1 cup (235 ml) water
1 teaspoon (5 ml) vanilla extract
2 tablespoons (26 g) sugar
3 cups (735 g) *Pure Plum Purée*, page 163
Juice of two oranges

1. In a medium saucepan over high heat, heat the water, vanilla, and sugar. After it comes to a small boil, reduce the heat to medium and let simmer for 5 to 7 minutes, until the liquid is reduced by one-fourth.

2. In a large bowl, combine the *Pure Plum Purée* and the orange juice.

3. Pour the sugar mixture over the plum mixture and combine.

4. Pour mixture in a deep-dish pan and freeze overnight. Scoop or scrape out frozen Italian ices for your family.

Lasagna Bolognese

17+ months

YIELD: 10 TO 12 SERVINGS

Lasagna is a great meal to let the little ones help with. They love laying out the noodles in the cooking dish, scooping big portions of the bolognese sauce, and digging in to the mozzarella cheese. I can even let River, who is 19 months, help me prepare this meal once it gets to the family assembly line. Children are far more capable than we give them credit for. The beauty of allowing our children to help us cook is that we not only pass down recipes to them, but we also we pass on cooking traditions. Cooking gives them fond food memories to carry with them into their adult lives.

One 9-ounce (255 g) package of lasagna noodles
2 cups (230 g) shredded mozzarella cheese, divided
2 cups (500 g) ricotta cheese
1 cup (100 g) grated Parmesan cheese
2 eggs, beaten
5 cups (1.25 kg) *Bolognese Textured Meal*, page 164
1 tablespoon (8 g) capers
1 cup (130 g) chopped carrots
1 cup (120 g) chopped zucchini

1. Preheat the oven to 350°F (180°C, or gas mark 4).
2. Boil the lasagna noodles according to the package directions. Drain and set aside.
3. In a large bowl, combine the cheeses with the two eggs. Save about ¼ cup (30 g) of the mozzarella cheese for topping the last layer.
4. In another bowl, combine the *Bolognese Textured Meal* with the capers, carrots, and zucchini. This is your sauce.
5. In a 9 x 13-inch (22.8 x 33 cm) baking dish, lay one-third of the lasagna noodles across the bottom of the pan.
6. Top with one-third of the sauce and one-third of the cheese. Repeat this process 3 times. Top the last layer with a little extra mozzarella cheese.
7. Cover with foil and bake for 30 minutes. Uncover and bake for an additional 10 minutes.
8. Let rest 15 to 20 minutes before slicing, so lasagna has time to firm up a bit. Serve warm.

Mozzarella, Tomato, and Basil Panini

15+ months

YIELD: 2 ADULT SERVINGS OR 4 KID SERVINGS

....

I love panini, and I have gotten my littlest baby, River, totally into them, too. I think a flavor-packed warm sandwich is the perfect lunch in the winter. An investment in a panini maker is so worth it— the sandwich options are endless and the taste always delivers.

4 slices of ciabatta bread
½ cup (125 g) *Hummus Purée* (page 166), divided
4 thin slices of fresh mozzarella cheese, cut from a whole round, divided
1 tomato, sliced in thin rounds, divided
8 large fresh basil leaves, divided
2 tablespoons (28 ml) balsamic vinegar, divided

1. Preheat panini press.
2. Spread the bread slices with the hummus, then assemble the sandwiches by layering two of the bread slices each with: a slice of the mozzarella, a few slices of tomatoes, 4 basil leaves, a tablespoon (15 ml) or so drizzle of balsamic vinegar, and one final slice of mozzarella. Place remaining slices of bread on top, hummus side down.
3. Carefully place the sandwiches on the press and cook until cheese is melted. This should take about 6 minutes (3 minutes per side if you prefer to turn your panini).
4. Serve warm.

Sausage and Corn Breakfast Bake

15+ months

YIELD: 8 TO 10 SERVINGS

....

This savory breakfast is hearty and so easy to make. We do big holiday breakfast gatherings, and I am always excited to see some savory choices available among all the sweet breakfast items. Being a busy mama, this recipe is one that I use on a regular basis.

½ pound (225 g) Italian sausage, casings removed
1½ cups (355 ml) whole milk
8 slices sourdough or brioche bread, cubed
1 cup (120 g) shredded cheddar cheese
1 cup (120 g) shredded Monterey jack cheese
11 eggs, beaten well
1 cup (245 g) *Bright Corn Purée*, page 167

1. Preheat the oven to 350° F (180° C, or gas mark 4).
2. In a medium sauté pan over medium-high heat, cook the sausage, break it up into bite sizes as it cooks, about 5 minutes.
3. When the meat is nicely browned and cooked, place it in a 9 x 13-inch (22.8 x 33 cm) dish.
4. In a large mixing bowl, combine the milk, bread, cheeses, eggs, and *Bright Corn Purée*.
5. Pour the mixture over the sausage.
6. Bake for 25 minutes covered, and then an additional 20 to 30 minutes uncovered.

Breakfast Waffles for Dinner

15+ months

YIELD: 6 TO 8 WAFFLES

We love having breakfast for dinner, and I love waffles, so this is the perfect meal. Serve these waffles with a side of pure maple syrup, and you will be in pure heaven! Note that you will need a waffle iron to create this dish.

1¾ cups (219 g) all-purpose flour
2 teaspoons (10 g) baking powder
½ teaspoon sea salt
1 teaspoon cinnamon
½ teaspoon ground nutmeg
1 teaspoon ground flaxseed
2 eggs, beaten
1 cup (235 ml) milk
½ teaspoon vanilla extract
½ cup (125 g) *Sweet Potato, Prosciutto, and Cheese Purée*, page 168
2 tablespoons (28 g) butter, for serving
½ cup (68 g) chopped pistachios, for serving
1 cup (340 g) pure maple syrup, for serving

1. Preheat waffle iron.
2. In a large bowl, combine the flour, baking powder, sea salt, cinnamon, nutmeg, and ground flaxseed.
3. In a separate bowl, whisk together the eggs with the milk and vanilla.
4. Fold in *Sweet Potato, Prosciutto, and Cheese Purée*. If the batter seems too thick, add more milk. It should be similar in consistency to pancake batter.
5. Spray waffle iron with a non-stick spray, if desired.
6. Ladle ½ cup (125 g) batter onto the waffle iron. Cook until the waffle is golden brown.
7. Serve hot topped with butter, pistachios, and maple syrup.

Sweet and Creamy Winter Ice Pops

13+ months

YIELD: 12 TO 15 ICE POPS

Even in the winter, ice pops are a favorite in my home. One of my kids' absolute favorite things to do is eat ice pops by a roaring fire. It's fun to look out over our snowy landscape from inside our cozy home, sucking on some immunity-boosting treats. Note: You will need some ice pop molds or a handful of small paper cups and wooden craft sticks to execute this recipe.

3 cups (750 g) *Cranberry, Pomegranate, and Greek Yogurt Purée*, page 169
1 whole pineapple, peeled and cut into chunks
¼ cup (85 g) honey

1. Purée all the ingredients in a blender or food processor.
2. Pour into individual paper cups or popsicle molds of your choice, and let freeze until solid.

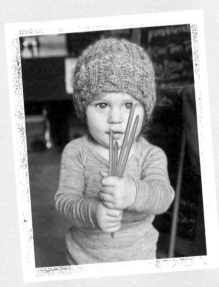

resources

Grocery and Specialty Food Items

RAW AGAVE NECTAR
www.madhavasweeteners.com

ORGANIC COCONUT SUGAR
www.azurestandard.com

WHOLESOME SWEETENERS
www.wholesomesweeteners.com

NATURAL FOOD COLORS
www.naturesflavors.com

FLOUR
www.kingarthurflour.com
www.fairhavenflour.com

EGGS (If you don't have a local farmers'
market, these are great eggs)
www.bornfreeeggs.com

LIQUID AMINOS
http://bragg.com

HEMP SEEDS & OTHER SUPER GRAINS
www.navitasnaturals.com

Cookware and Container Products

LIFE WITHOUT PLASTIC
(My friend Jay's amazing store)
http://lifewithoutplastic.com/

LODGE CAST IRON COOKWARE
www.lodgemfg.com

KLEAN KANTEEN
www.kleankanteen.com

KUHN RIKON
www.kuhnrikon.com

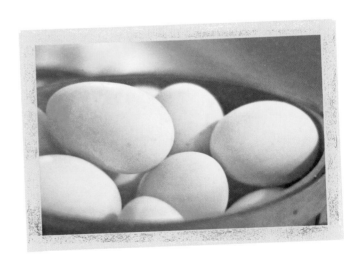

about the author

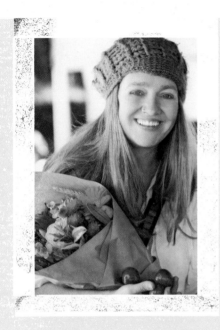

Anni Daulter is a family living lifestyle expert, professional cook, and advocate of sustainable living. She is the author of *Organically Raised: Conscious Cooking for Babies and Toddlers, Ice Pop Joy, The Organic Family Cookbook, Naturally Fun Parties for Kids*, and *Sacred Pregnancy*.

Anni was the founder and operator of Bohemian Baby, a fresh organic baby food company, for three years, where she developed all recipes and branding for the company. She is currently a healthy eating expert for the nonprofit organization Healthy Child Healthy World, an ambassador for Nordic Naturals, and is also the resident baby/toddler food expert for Hot Moms Club, City Mommy, Citibabes NY, Mindful Mama, Green Moms, and Macaroni Kid.

Anni lives in Pennsylvania with her husband and four children. Please visit her at www.annidaulter.com and www.sacredpregnancy.com.

about the photographer

Elena Rego is a writer and photographer committed to creating work that highlights conscious living. Deeply drawn to food and the cultural patterns we all share with one another across the dinner table, she has created a food blog at www.foodpractice.com, where she explores recipes, mealtime rituals, sustainable slow food, and rich enticing food photography.

Elena is currently writing a book on the basics of food practice and enjoying her new home on the lush island of Maui with her beloved and their dog.

acknowledgments

I want to thank so many people who helped turn this book into a reality. Cookbooks are tough to make, and there are a lot of folks that make one come together. This is my sixth book in three years. I cannot believe that all these folks have come together to help make all this happen time and time again. Thank you.

As always, I want to thank my family. My husband, Tim, for his endless ability to support me and my projects. That well runs very deep, and I am so grateful for all you do for me and our family. My kiddos, Lotus, Zoe, Bodhi, and River, who have taught me virtues of patience, understanding, and the deepest love in the world. You all are the purée in my cupcake!

To my mom, I love you so much. Thank you for being proud of me and my work. Thank you to my agent on this book, Sally Ekus.

To my editor, Amanda Waddell, thanks for hanging in there and helping to create such a fun and inspired book. Thanks also to all the design folks and line editors at Fair Winds for making the book so gorgeous!

Elena—wow! We did it. That was a crazy week, and I am so glad that we have come back together to create again. Remember Spiral Musings? We have come a long way since then. I adore you and honor you as a soul sister.

Cari Ellen—thanks for your help with the last few shots. We appreciate your work! See www.cariellen.dphoto.com to see more of her work.

Thank you to Gina Sabatella (www.sabatellafoto.com), Alexandra DeFurio (www.defuriophotography.com), Tnah DiDanto (www.bellafacciafoto.com), and Denne Boring (www.etsy.com/people/DenneAlise) for sharing your talent.

Ellen—thank you so much for taking me under your Kimberton wing and stepping into my crazy world and helping me so much. Bringing us lunch that day at Bobby's saved us, and staying in the kitchen all night helping me prep was above and beyond. You are a great friend, and I am so glad we met.

Karen, from the Food for Thought program at Kimberton Waldorf School, thank you for allowing me to use your kitchen space and for hanging out to cut veggies with me so I would not have to be alone. Your program of making organic, fresh lunches for the whole school every day with locally sourced foods should be modeled by every school in America. Check out Food for Thought at www.kimberton.org/academics/food-for-thought.

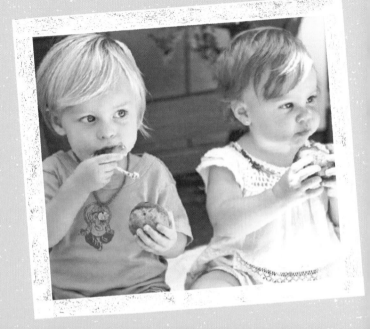

Thank you to all my models! Lotus, Bodhi, River, Ceila, Anthony, Koa, Ewen, Estelle, Taj, Ryan, Lake, Jude, Collin, Samantha, and Faith.

Thank you Alan Moore from Folk Art, for creating such a special and unique art piece to open this book up with. Those amazing spoons and vintage knives bring the piece to life. I love that this book has an original folk art piece! Please check out more folk art at www.etsy.com/shop/sweettatersjunkyard.

Thank you Jennifer Babcock from The Funki Little Frog for making those great signs for the book. I love the "you are the purée in my cupcake" sign. Your work is incredible, and I appreciate it so much. These special touches make the book so much fun. Please check out more of Jennifer's work at www.etsy.com/shop/TheFunkiLittleFrog.

Thank you Cara Corey from Mary Marie Knits, for the use of the big orange pouf for our photos. Your work is fun and delightful and brightens up life. Please check out Cara's work at www.etsy.com/shop/marymarieknits.

Thank you Sarah Hepworth from Little Miss Loolies for the use of your adorable balls of fun for the photo shoots. Your work is delightful. Please check her out at www.etsy.com/shop/littlemissloolies.

Thank you Cara Graver from Cob Studio for allowing us to use your space to shoot. Your amazing studio is magical and wondrous. Please visit the Cob Studio at www.thecobstudio.com.

Thank you Bobby at Frog Hollow Farm for sharing your gorgeous chickens and amazing home with us for the photo shoot! You are a good friend, and I adore your Ben as he has rapidly become my second teenage boy! Visit Frog Hollow Farm from Phoenixville, Pennsylvania on Facebook.

Thank you Seven Stars Farm for allowing us to meet Pearl and the other new baby calves and take pictures of your precious cows. Your yogurt and cream is amazing, and I feel so blessed to have you in my backyard! Check out Seven Stars Farm at www.sevenstarsfarm.com.

Thank you Susan for allowing us to use your guest house to cook all day and shoot at your farm space. We miss you guys.

index